Calcium and the Heart

Calcium and the Heart

*Proceedings of the meeting of the European Section
of the International Study Group for Research in Cardiac
Metabolism held at the Institute of Cardiology, London,
on 6 September, 1970*

Edited by
P. HARRIS
*Institute of Cardiology
London, England*

L. OPIE
*Department of Medicine
University of Cape Town
and Groote Schuur Hospital,
South Africa*

 1971

ACADEMIC PRESS · London and New York

ACADEMIC PRESS INC. (LONDON) LTD.
Berkeley Square House
Berkeley Square
London, W1X 6BA

U.S. Edition published by
ACADEMIC PRESS INC.
111 Fifth Avenue
New York, New York 10003

Copyright © 1971 By ACADEMIC PRESS INC. (LONDON) LTD.

All Rights Reserved
No part of this book may be reproduced in any form by photostat, microfilm, or any other means, without written permission from the publishers

Library of Congress Catalog Card Number: 70-153539
ISBN: 0-12-326950-4

Printed in Great Britain by
BIDDLES LTD., MARTYR ROAD, GUILDFORD, SURREY

CONTRIBUTORS

A. FLECKENSTEIN, Physiological Institute, University of Freiburg, Germany

HARRIET L. GOODHART, The Mount Sinai School of Medicine of The City University, New York 10029, U.S.A.

PHILLIP J. GOODHART, The Mount Sinai School of Medicine of The City University, New York 10029, U.S.A.

ARNOLD M. KATZ, The Mount Sinai School of Medicine of The City University, New York 10029, U.S.A.

W. KÜBLER, Department of Cardiology, University of Dusseldorf, Germany

N. C. R. MERRILLEES, Department of Anatomy, University of Melbourne, Parkville, Victoria, Australia

WINIFRED G. NAYLER, Baker Medical Research Institute, Melbourne, Australia

ROBERT E. OLSON, School of Medicine, St. Louis University, St. Louis, Missouri 63104, U.S.A.

ARNOLD SCHWARTZ, Division of Myocardial Biology, Baylor College of Medicine, Houston, Texas 77025, U.S.A.

E. A. SHINEBOURNE, Institute of Cardiology, University of London, England

PREFACE

Molecular and cellular studies have come perhaps later to Cardiology than to many other branches of Medicine. Traditionally the cardiac physiologist has been concerned with the engineering properties of a pump, but recent years have seen a growing interest in the more intimate working of the myocardial cell on which the overt mechanical properties of the heart largely depend. This logical extension of interest has been encouraged by those technical advances in studying the structure and chemical properties of subcellular components which have revolutionised biology as a whole. Equally, the surgical mechanical solution of many cardiac abnormalities has revealed to the clinician the importance of the function of the myocardium itself.

To his intuitive vision of the working of the myocardial cell, the physiologist or physician brings images from mechanical engineering — ropes and springs and engines. Ropes he can see, alternating thick and thin ones, but to grasp the engine needs a new set of symbols, those of the biochemist. Now he finds himself in a world of thermodynamics and enzyme kinetics. In this complex world, one simple substance seems to have an ubiquitous importance — calcium.

For the clinical properties of calcium ions, the cardiologist already has some respect, keeping solutions of calcium salts at hand in his coronary care unit. This book is concerned with the intimate activities of calcium ions within the heart muscle cell — their distribution, their rhythmic sequestration by sarcoplasmic reticulum, their flux across the cell wall membrane, their specific effects on the contractile proteins and the pathological effects of abnormal accumulations. It is believed that the bringing together of all of these aspects of calcium metabolism in the cell will be of help not only to those working on individual aspects of the subject, but also to those physiologists and clinicians to whom the myocardium is important.

The book arises out of the 1970 meeting of the European Section of the International Study Group for Research in Cardiac Metabolism at the Institute of Cardiology, London. The contributors, each distinguished in an aspect of myocardial calcium metabolism, were asked to provide a survey of their subject in addition to presenting recent work. In this way an up-to-date review of the whole field was presented, the success of which was such that it was felt that its publication would be welcome to a wider audience.

May, 1971   P. HARRIS

CONTENTS

INTRODUCTION ROBERT E. OLSON   1
 I. Calcium and the beating heart   2
 II. Contractile proteins and contraction in vitro   4
 III. Relaxation and relaxing factors   7
 IV. Excitation-contraction coupling   10
 V. The application of fundamental knowledge to the problem of cardiac failure   14
  References   19

CELLULAR EXCHANGE OF CALCIUM
  WINIFRED G. NAYLER AND N.C.R. MERRILLEES   24
 I. Introduction   24
 II. Distribution of Ca^{2+} in cardiac muscle   25
 III. Calcium exchange associated with the action potential   35
 IV. Calcium exchange and the activation of contraction   40
 V. Membrane depolarization and the activation of contraction   46
 VI. Conclusion   54
  References   56

CALCIUM AND THE SARCOPLASMIC RETICULUM
  ARNOLD SCHWARTZ   66
 I. Introduction and history   66
 II. Materials and methods   76
 III. Results   76
 IV. Discussion   87
  References   90

CALCIUM AND THE MITOCHONDRIA
  W. KÜBLER AND E.A. SHINEBOURNE   93
  References   115

CALCIUM AND THE CARDIAC CONTRACTILE PROTEINS
ARNOLD M. KATZ AND PHILIP J. AND HARRIET L. GOODHART   124
   References   134

SPECIFIC INHIBITORS AND PROMOTERS OF CALCIUM ACTION IN THE EXCITATION-CONTRACTION COUPLING OF HEART MUSCLE AND THEIR ROLE IN THE PREVENTION OR PRODUCTION OF MYOCARDIAL LESIONS   A. FLECKENSTEIN   135

  I. Inhibitors of excitation-contraction coupling   138
  II. Promoters of excitation-contraction coupling   151
  III. Intracellular Ca overload leading to high-energy phosphate deficiency as an etiological factor in the production of myocardial fibre necroses   157
    References   182

Author Index   189

Subject Index   196

INTRODUCTION*

ROBERT E. OLSON

Department of Biochemistry, St. Louis University,
School of Medicine, St. Louis, Mo. 63104, U.S.A.

I was pleased, and at the same time filled with some misgivings, when Professor Harris asked me to introduce this symposium on the subject of **Calcium and the Heart.** It is always a delicate task to introduce, with just the right brevity and emphasis, a subject which is to be considered in depth by a panel of experts. If one neglects the important historical developments leading up to the present state of knowledge, the panelists are annoyed because it costs them time to fill in these essential facts. If, on the other hand, one devotes too much time to the current research effort, then there is consternation among the panel members because some of the punch has been taken out of their presentations. Nonetheless, an audience such as is assembled today, composed of medical students, practising physicians, and physiologists, not specialists in this field, generally appreciates some overlap and

---

*Paper delivered at the Meeting of The International Study Group for Research in Cardiac Metabolism, September 6, 1970, London, England.

repetition in the presentations. So in this rectangular strait, a sort of double Scylla and Charybdis, I shall do my best to give some historical perspective to the subject of this symposium, which I consider a very important current research frontier in cardiology. I shall, furthermore, emphasize the biochemical evolution of this problem since my own work has dealt principally with biochemical aspects of the problem.

I should like to consider five main topics which have become coherent areas of study during the development of this subject. They are: (1) the rôle of calcium in supporting the beat of the intact heart, (2) the identification of the contractile proteins and the recreation of the contractile event in vitro, (3) the investigations leading to an understanding of relaxation, (4) theories of excitation-contraction coupling, and (5) application of this fundamental knowledge to the problem of cardiac failure.

I. CALCIUM AND THE BEATING HEART

The rôle of calcium in normal cardiac physiology was first appreciated by Sidney Ringer,[51] who reported that ionic calcium is required to sustain the beat of the heart in vitro. At that time, and for many years thereafter, this observation was interpreted to mean that the cardiac cell membrane was calcium-sensitive as are, indeed, other mammalian cell membranes. That there was an unusual dependence of heart muscle upon external calcium did not become evident until later. In 1907 Locke and Rosenheim[38] reported that the action potential of the isolated perfused heart persisted long after contractility diminished, suggesting that

INTRODUCTION

calcium played another rôle in the heart, in addition to maintaining membrane competence. This view was greatly strengthened by Heilbrun and Wiercinski[26] who showed that microinjections of calcium into muscle cells would initiate contraction. Thus it was evident as early as 1947 that excitation-contraction coupling involved (or could involve) calcium ions. Subsequently, other investigators[45] observed that peak tension in the frog heart was dependent upon external calcium in the range of 0-4 mM, and that polarization of the cardiac membrane was less dependent upon calcium than upon sodium, potassium and proton concentrations.

In 1959, Bianchi and Shanes[6] showed that the calcium uptake, studied with ^{45}Ca, increased progressively in skeletal muscle during repetitive contractions. Subsequently, Winegrad and Shanes[57], Niedergierke,[46] Langer,[35] and Grossman and Furchgott[20] showed that the same phenomenon can be demonstrated in cardiac muscle, and that in this tissue the resting uptake of calcium of 0.009 μmoles/sq cm/sec could be augmented with repetitive contractions to 0.11 μmoles/sq cm/sec, or a 12-fold increase in calcium entry. The classical Bowditch staircase, a plot of increased contractility with repetitive stimulation, is now thought to be due to accumulating intracellular calcium.[45] All the evidence points to a much greater dependence by cardiac muscle upon external calcium as a source of internal calcium, than in skeletal muscle, where contractility is regulated almost solely from internal stores of calcium.

II. CONTRACTILE PROTEINS AND CONTRACTION IN VITRO

The two major contractile proteins of muscle, myosin and actin, were discovered respectively by H.H. Weber in 1934[56] and Albert Szent-Gyorgyi in 1942.[2] Myosin is a fibrous protein with a molecular weight of 500,000 and dimensions of 1500 x 30 Å. It has a calcium stimulated ATP-ase activity which is almost completely inhibited by physiological concentrations of potassium ions.[15] As shown in Fig. 1, it consists of two heavy chains, of molecular weight 220,000, that traverse the entire length of the molecule and three light chains which are associated with the bulbous head averaging about 20,000 in molecular weight. One light chain is removed with reagents that combine with sulfhydril groups and two are made labile by alkali. The ATP-ase activity of myosin, and its actin-combining activity, are associated with the head of the molecule and are dependent upon the presence and integrity of the light chains.[39] Short trypsin digestion produces two fragments, light meromyosin (LMM) and heavy meromyosin (HMM), both double helical structures, which account for all but a few percent of the nitrogen of the myosin molecule. As shown further in Fig. 1, subfragment 1 of HMM can be obtained by further controlled digestion of HMM. The two heads of myosin can be seen in the electron microscope. Myosins from different muscle types (red and white skeletal muscle and cardiac muscle) are identical in size, shape and physical properties, but vary in their intrinsic ATP-ase activity.[3,42] They may be regarded as a family of isoenzymes.

Actin, the second major contractile protein of muscle, was

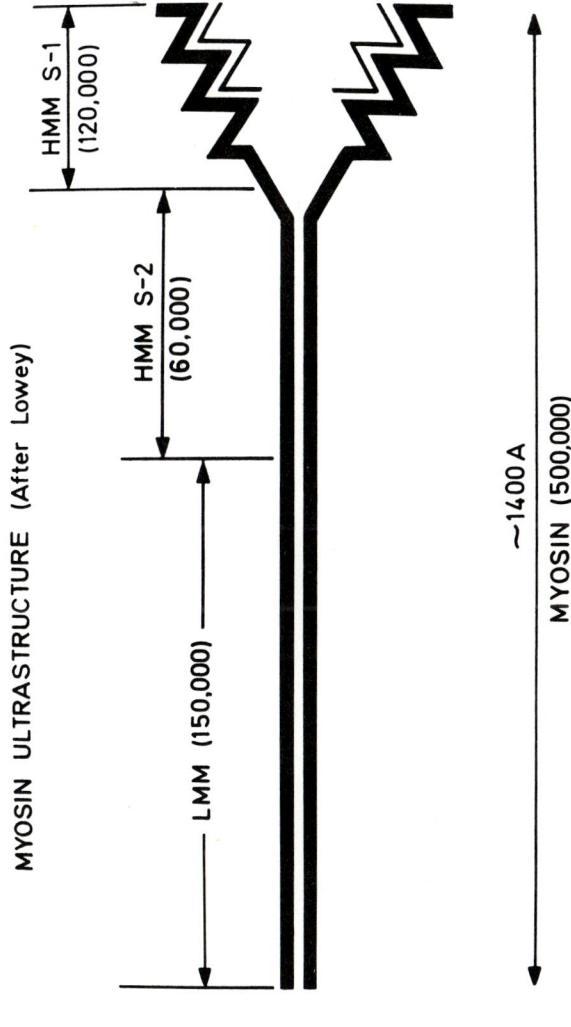

Fig. 1. Myosin ultrastructure (after Lowey et al.[39]). LMM = light meromyosin; HMM = heavy meromyosin; HMM S-1 and S-2 = subfragments of HMM containing the ATP-ase center, and remainder of the molecule respectively.

discovered[2] by prolonged extraction of muscle with hypertonic salt solutions which yielded much more viscous preparations containing myosin combined with actin. These were found to dissociate in the presence of ATP into myosin and polymerized actin (F-actin) which had a molecular weight of the order of 1,500,000. In acetone powders of muscle, actin exists in monomeric form (G-actin), a small globular protein with a molecular weight of 70,000. In the presence of ATP and Mg ions, G-actin polymerizes to F-actin. In F-actin the monomers appear to be spheres with a diameter of 55 Å.

Albert Szent-Gyorgyi showed in 1942[2] that at ionic strengths less than 0.3, similar to the intracellular milieu, F-actin and myosin combined to form a colloidal gel with a high viscosity and a molecular weight greater than 20,000,000. In the presence of magnesium ion and ATP, the gel was found to contract (syneresis) and split ATP. The phenomenon of the syneresis of actomyosin, associated with a magnesium-stimulated ATP-ase, has been employed since as an in vitro model for muscle contraction.

In 1954, studies by A. F. Huxley and R. Niedergierke[27] and H. Huxley and J. Hansen[28] by phase and electron microscopy, respectively, revealed the true nature of the ultrastructure of muscle, and the intracellular distribution of the contractile proteins. These workers observed that two types of filament exist in the myofibril. The thicker ones, about 150 Å in diameter, which coincide with the A-bands of the sarcomere, are composed of an orderly array of myosin molecules (about 400 of them) with an axis of symmetry in the center of the filament, so that the sense of orientation is opposite in the two halves. The LMM portions of these myosin molecules form the backbone of the filament, whereas the HMM (head) portions projected from the axis of the filament. Each thick filament was surrounded by six thin filaments which arise from the Z-line structure at each end of the sarcomere (1-2 microns apart) and project toward the center of the sarcomere. It is now known that the thin filaments are composed of a double helix of F-actin molecules, about 100 Å in diameter plus an array of regulatory proteins which will be discussed subsequently. Along the zone of overlap, interaction between the projecting myosin cross bridges and the actin molecules can occur. In fact, shortening of the sarcomere during muscular contraction was demonstrated by the two Huxley teams (supra vide) to occur without a change in the A-band length by simple sliding of the thin filaments. This involves the making and breaking of many actomyosin bridges during shortening, presumably with the splitting of one ATP molecule at the instant of each cross bridge interaction. Thus, actomyosin formation in living muscle is a highly oriented and repetitive process.[29]

III. RELAXATION AND RELAXING FACTORS

It is perhaps not surprising that our knowledge of the nature of the regulatory events in contractility of muscle came from a systematic study of the phenomenon of relaxation. In 1951, Marsh,[40] working in Kenneth Bailey's laboratory in Cambridge, observed that supernatant fraction obtained during the preparation of myofibrils from muscle contained a factor which would reverse syneresis. Associated with this redispersion of the actomyosin gel, was a reduction in actomyosin ATP-ase activity. The active compound in the supernatant fraction appeared to be a protein or complex of proteins, and the experiments were originally interpreted to indicate that a protein in the cytosol combined with actomyosin and inhibited its ATP-ase activity. Several soluble enzymes were suggested as relaxing factors.[4] Subsequent studies by Ebashi and his colleagues at the University of Tokyo,[33] however, demonstrated that the 'relaxing factor' was not soluble, as had been claimed by some, but was granular, sedimentable at 18,000 x g for one hour, and possessed of ATP-ase activity. In fact, this granular fraction was identified with a similar fraction described in 1948 by Kielley and Meyerhof[31] as a non-mitochondrial, non-myofibrillar, membranous ATP-ase whose enzyme activity was lost upon incubation with phospholipase C. In the meantime, Bozler[7] and Watanabe[52] demonstrated that ethylenediamine tetracetic acid (EDTA), a chelating agent for calcium, magnesium and other divalent ions, could induce relaxation in glycerinated muscle fibers. This finding led Perry and Grey[49] to test the effect of EDTA upon 'relaxation', i.e. inhibition of ATP-ase activity of myofibrils and actomyosin gels. They observed that the ATP-ase activity of myofibrils and native actomyosin preparations were uniformly inhibited by EDTA and suggested that some divalent ion was involved in the contraction-relaxation cycle. This conclusion led to two pertinent questions: (1) Does the actomyosin ATP-ase have a requirement for calcium? (2) Can the granules of Kielley and Meyerhof concentrate calcium, i.e. remove it from the sarcoplasm?

The first question was answered by Annemarie Weber, working at Columbia University in 1959.[53] She showed that the inhibitory effects of EDTA upon myofibrillar ATP-ase was to remove traces of calcium, and that the ATP-ase activity of these myofibrils could be restored by the addition of calcium, the apparent K_m for calcium being about 10^{-6} M. She suggested, as a corollary, that the 'relaxing granules' of Marsh might remove calcium, and thus induce relaxation.

The second question, relating to the calcium-pumping ability of the Kielly-Meyerhof-Marsh granules, was answered in the affirmative in 1961 by Hasselbach and Makinose,[25] working at the Max Planck Institute in Heidelberg. They demonstrated that these granules contained an ATP-dependent calcium pump which could concentrate cytoplasmic calcium 500 times. In the presence of oxalate, a permeant anion which served as an intragranular trap for calcium, the concentration difference could reach 6000 times, with a reduction in the external calcium to 0.1 μM, more than sufficient to inhibit myofibrillar ATP-ase and thus induce relaxation. In 1962, Ebashi and Lipmann[14] independently confirmed the work of Hasselbach and Makinose and, further, showed by electron microscopy that the Ca-pumping granules were, in fact, part of the endoplasmic reticulum of the muscle cell. They demonstrated that discrete vesicles existed in their preparation which appeared to be the sites of calcium concentration.

IV. EXCITATION-CONTRACTION COUPLING

With the publication of these important observations on the rôle of calcium in regulating the state of contraction or relaxation of myofibrils, much speculation took place about the mechanism of excitation-contraction coupling, i.e. the link between neuromuscular excitation and myofibrillar shortening. The earlier proposal of Morales et al.[41] which postulated that electrostatic forces generated by the action potential caused deformation of the actomyosin system, had to be abandoned in favor of a more chemical hypothesis. In 1963, Robert Davies at the University of Pennsylvania[10] proposed that calcium ions released from longitudinal tubules linked the heads of myosin molecules to actin combining sites in the sliding filament model of the Huxleys, and produced an electrostatic gradient which caused the cross bridges to shorten and the filaments to move along one another. The novelty of this idea produced an interesting debate for several years, but again was abandoned when it was demonstrated by Ebashi[12] that the regulatory protein binding calcium was distinct from myosin. Of the early investigators of muscle function, Bailey's views of regulation of contraction were most prophetic. In 1948[1] he discovered a new, relatively small (molecular weight 70,000) protein from the thin filaments of muscle, which he named tropomyosin. It was a long, slender, highly helical protein, which he demonstrated could combine with actin and which he speculated might regulate the reaction between myosin and actin. Although more recent studies have shown that the calcium protein is also distinct from tropomyosin, tropomyosin is required as an

INTRODUCTION

integral part of the regulatory system.

The search for the calcium regulatory protein of muscle can be traced to observations made by Perry and Grey[50] at Cambridge in 1956. These investigators reported that the ATP-ase activity of various actomyosin preparations was affected differently by EDTA. If native actomyosin was prepared directly from muscle extracts without rigorous purification, its Mg-activated ATP-ase was invariably reduced by EDTA. On the other hand, 'synthetic' actomyosins made by combining purified myosin with purified actin frequently did not show such an inhibition of ATP-ase when treated with EDTA. In 1961, A. Weber and Winicur[54] confirmed these observations and concluded that calcium removal by EDTA or EGTA did not **directly** affect the interaction between actin and myosin. They observed, furthermore, that the loss of calcium sensitivity was a function of actin and not myosin purification. Presumably, some regulatory protein, associated with actin, was being removed in the calcium insensitive preparations.

In 1964, Ebashi's group in Tokyo[11] reported that actin prepared according to Straub, which contained tropomyosin, could restore calcium sensitivity to insensitive synthetic actomyosin. They also showed that crude tropomyosin prepared by Bailey's method contained another protein which they named 'troponin'. A year later Ebashi and Kodama[12, 13] reported the isolation of troponin and identified it as the calcium-binding protein responsible for the calcium sensitivity of native myofibrils. It appears to be a globular protein with a molecular weight of 45,000, a calcium binding capacity of 2 moles per mole, and a binding constant of

10^{-6} M. The native tropomyosin prepared by Bailey's method was shown to contain two molecules of tropomyosin and one of troponin, representing a segment of the tropomyosin-troponin complex present in the thin filament (Fig. 2). Recent work on the substructure of troponin by Hartshorne and Mueller[22-24] has revealed that troponin is composed of two dissimilar subunits, troponin A (molecular weight 18,000) and troponin B (molecular weight 30,000). Troponin A is the calcium-binding subunit and binds 2 moles calcium per mole of protein. Troponin B is inhibitory to actomyosin ATP-ase in the absence of troponin A. In the presence of troponin A, the inhibitory action of the B-subunit is relieved. These investigators also demonstrated that troponin and tropomyosin form a 1:1 complex which augments the regulatory effects of troponin upon actomyosin ATP-ase, i.e. in the presence of tropomyosin, troponin exerts maximum activation of actomyosin ATP-ase in the presence of calcium and a maximum inhibition of ATP-ase in the absence of calcium.

It appears that, as shown in Fig. 2, the troponin-tropomyosin complex lies in the sulcus of the double helix formed by intertwining F-actin molecules. The arrangement of the proteins composing the thick and thin filaments accounts for the 400 Å periodicity of muscle. The tropomyosin-troponin complex is 400 Å long; the half period of the actin double helix is 370 Å, and the rotation of myosin heads in the thick filament brings heads in to the same plane roughly every 429 Å.[29] What remains to be learned is the mechanism by which the tropomyosin-troponin system regulates the actin-myosin interaction. The presence of calcium could

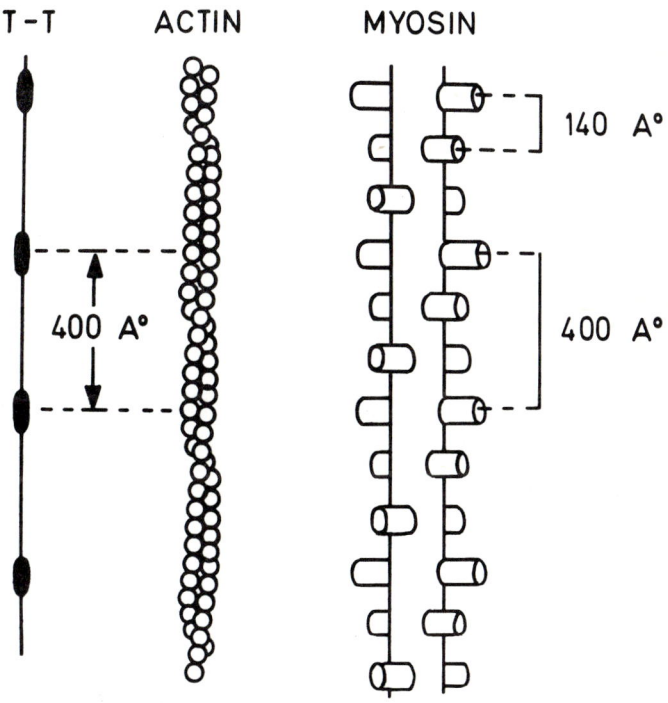

Fig. 2. Ultrastructure of thick and thin filaments. The thin filament is a double helix of F-actin in the sulcus of which lies the troponin-tropomyosin (T-T) system. Myosin heads project from the thick filament at regular intervals with a spacing of 60°.

conceivably change the conformation of troponin to the extent
required to alter the double helical arrangement of actin molecules and hence the reactivity of these molecules to projecting
myosin heads. Further studies of this fundamental problem will
be awaited with great interest.

In summary, excitation of the contractile mechanism begins
with the movement of the action potential of the muscle cell
membrane down the invaginating T-system to the associated
longitudinal system. The longitudinal reticulum, which contains
sequestered calcium, is depolarized, its membrane becomes
permeable to calcium, and calcium is released into the sarcoplasm.
In cardiac muscle, appreciable amounts also enter from the
extracellular space. This calcium diffuses into the myofibrils,
combines with troponin (which in the calcium-free state inhibits
myosin-actin interaction), and releases this inhibition. Actin
subunits of F-actin combine with myosin, ATP-ase activity
appears, ATP is split, and the thin filaments move along the thick
ones, with resultant shortening of the myofibril. As the intracellular free calcium rises from 10^{-7} M to values as high as
10^{-5} M, the longitudinal system pumps the calcium back into its
lacunae, and relaxation occurs.

V. THE APPLICATION OF FUNDAMENTAL KNOWLEDGE TO THE PROBLEM OF CARDIAC FAILURE

Any comprehensive knowledge of pathologic physiology is
predicated upon an understanding of normal physiology. These
developments in the field of fundamental muscle physiology are of

intense interest to physicians concerned with the management of disorders of muscle. Of particular importance to cardiologists is the problem of congestive heart failure.

Clinical heart failure has many etiologies, ranging from those conditions such as anoxia, coenzyme lack, and hormonal changes that limit energy production (ATP synthesis) and disorders arising from chronic mechanical overload or inflammatory disease which appear to inhibit energy utilization (ATP hydrolysis).[16,47] What may be developing on the tide of new knowledge about excitation-contraction coupling and the rôle of calcium is the possibility that many forms of cardiac failure may have as a common thread of pathogenesis, a disturbance in excitation-contraction coupling. They may, therefore, be regarded as disorders of regulation dependent upon the interplay of highly specialized membranes and macromolecular systems.

The basic physiology of excitation-contraction coupling in cardiac muscle is similar to that demonstrated for skeletal muscle as shown in Fig. 3. It appears that entry of calcium from the external medium plays a somewhat more important rôle in controlling the intracellular Ca concentration than in skeletal muscle, as has been mentioned earlier. The cardiac sarcoplasmic reticulum, although not as abundant as in skeletal muscle, has an active calcium pump, somewhat more labile and less energetic in vitro than skeletal muscle, but seemingly adequate for its rôle in vivo.[9,30,55] The suggestion by Patriarca and Carafoli[48] that mitochondria play a greater rôle in calcium metabolism in heart muscle is opposed by other data[32] that the

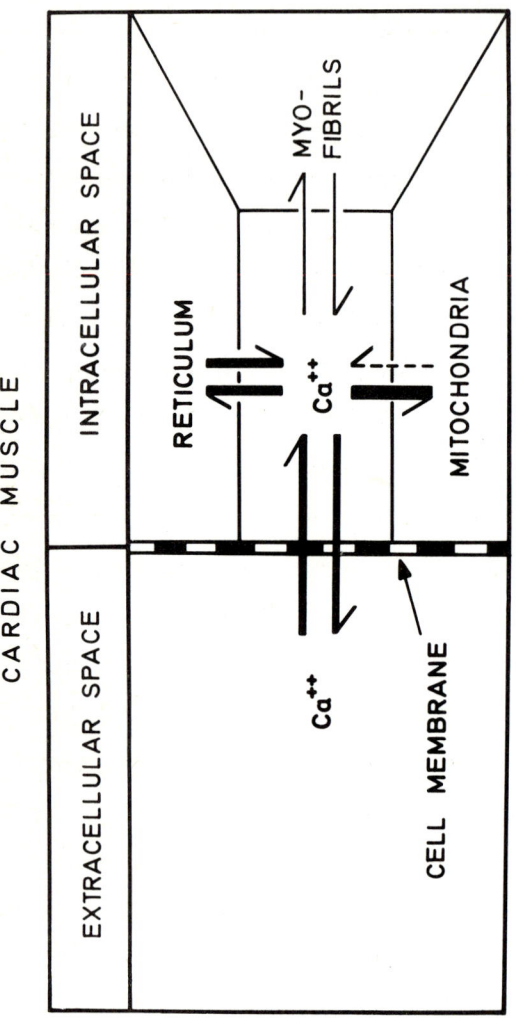

Fig. 3. Excitation-contraction coupling in cardiac muscle.

rate of uptake, and particularly release of calcium by heart mitochondria, is not sufficient for the task. The affinity of cardiac myofibrils for calcium seems to be the same as for skeletal muscle although their intrinsic ATP-ase activity is lower.[44]

A number of reports have appeared since 1966 attempting to relate disorders of cardiac contraction to an altered calcium flux, and more particularly a failure of the cardiac calcium pump. In 1966, Brigg's group at the University of Pittsburgh[8,34] observed that amytal, a barbiturate which can induce failure in isolated heart preparations, and depress cardiac function in mammals in situ, would depress calcium uptake by vesicles from dog myocardium, an effect which was reversed by ouabain. Subsequently this same group[17] reported that microsomes isolated from spontaneously failing isolated perfused hearts showed a modest (27%) fall in calcium accumulation in the presence of oxalate, which was also prevented by digitalis. On the other hand, Lee and Choi[37] observed that ouabain inhibited the uptake of calcium from the reticulum of normal dog hearts, and reasoned that this inhibition of uptake would give a positive inotropic effect by virtue of more intracellular calcium. They subsequently observed that severe anoxia had a similar effect.[36] Harigaya and Schwartz[21] observed that the calcium uptake of reticulum from failing human hearts, made available at the time of transplantation, was lower than demonstrated by preparations from other mammals with similar metabolic rates. Muir,[43] in my laboratory, has observed that isolated rat hearts perfused without substrate develop cardiac failure in about 30 minutes. Coincident with this he found a fall in calcium binding to the reticulum (Ca uptake without oxalate) although changes in calcium uptake in the presence of oxalate were not observed until two hours. Finally, Gertz et al.[18] have recently reported an alteration in the rate of calcium pumping by the reticulum of hearts from Syrian hamsters afflicted with hereditary cardiomyopathy. All of these reports suggest, but do not as yet establish, the conclusion that alterations in excitation-contraction coupling may be crucial for the development of cardiac failure in mammals. The mechanism of the action of digitalis is still clouded by controversy and contradictory experiments, but the idea that its therapeutic action is linked to its inhibition of the Na/K-dependent ATP-ase is gaining ground.[5,19] Calcium extrusion from cells is thought to depend upon the sodium pump; under the influence of digitalis, thus, intracellular calcium would tend to accumulate, particularly in the heart which has a large movement of calcium across its cell membrane.

I hope this introduction has set the stage properly for the presentations by Drs. Nayler, Schwartz, Kübler, Katz and Fleckenstein that will bring us all up to date on the subject of calcium and the heart.

References

1. Bailey, K. (1948). Tropomyosin: a new asymmetric protein component of the muscle fibril. Biochem. J., **43**, 271.

2. Banga, I. and Szent-Gyorgi, A. (1941-42). Preparation and properties of myosin A and B. In 'Studies from the Institute of Medical Chemistry, University of Szeged, Basle', vol. I.

3. Barany, M., Conover, T.E., Schliselfeld, L.H., Gaetjens, E. and Goffart, M. (1967). Relation of properties of isolated myosin to those of intact muscle of the cat and sloth. J. Biochem., **2**, 156.

4. Bendall, J.R. (1954). The relaxing effect of myokinase on muscle fibers: its identity with the 'Marsh' factor. Proc. Roy. Soc., Series B, **142**, 409.

5. Besch, H.R., Allen, J.C., Glick, G. and Schwartz, A. (1970). Correlation between the inotropic action of ouabain and its effects on subcellular enzyme systems from canine myocardium. J. Pharmacol., **171**, 1.

6. Bianchi, C.P. and Shanes, A.M. (1959). Calcium influx in skeletal muscle at rest, during octurity, and during potassium contraction. J. gen. Physiol., **42**, 803.

7. Bozler, E. (1954). Relaxation in extracted muscle fibers. J. gen. Physiol., **38**, 53.

8. Briggs, F.N., Gertz, E.W. and Hess, M.L. (1966) Calcium uptake by cardiac vesicles: Inhibition by amytal and reversal by ouabain. Biochem. Z., **345**, 122.

9. Carsten, M.E. (1964). The cardiac calcium pump. Proc. nat. Acad. Sci., Wash., **52**, 1456.

10. Davies, R.E. (1963). A molecular theory of muscle contraction: Calcium dependent contraction with hydrogen bond formation plus ATP-dependent extensions of part of the myosin actin cross bridges. Nature, Lond., **199**, 1068.

11 Ebashi, S. and Ebashi, F. (1964). A new protein component participating in the superprecipitation of myosin B. J. Biochem., **55**, 604.

12 Ebashi, S. and Kodama, A. (1965). A new protein factor promoting aggregation of tropomyosin. J. Biochem., **58**, 107.

13 Ebashi, S., Ebashi, F. and Kodama, A. (1967). Troponin as the Ca^{++} receptive protein in the contractile system. J. Biochem., **62**, 137.

14 Ebashi, S. and Lipmann, F. (1962). Adenosine triphosphate linked concentration of calcium ions in a particulate fraction of rabbit muscle. J. Cell Biol., **14**, 389.

15 Engelhardt, A. and Ljubimova, J. (1939). Myosin adenosinetriphosphatase. Nature, Lond., **144**, 668.

16 Fleckenstein, A. (1964). Herzstoffwechsel bei Koronarverschluss und Herzstillstand. In 'Herzinsufficienz, Hemodynamik und Stoffwechsel', p. 221. Thieme, Stuttgart.

17 Gertz, E.W., Hess, M.L., Lain, R.F. and Briggs, F.N. (1967). Activity of the vesicular calcium pump in the spontaneously failing heart-lung preparation. Circ. Res., **20**, 477.

18 Gertz, E.W., Stam, A.C. and Sonnenblick, E.H. (1970). A quantitative and qualitative defect in the sarcoplasmic reticulum in hereditary cardiomyopathy of Syrian hamsters. Biochem. Biophys. Res. Com., **40**, 746.

19 Glynn, I. (1964). The action of cardiac glycosides on ion movements. Pharmacol. Rev., **16**, 381.

20 Grossman, A. and Furchgott, R.F. (1964). The effects of various drugs on calcium exchange in the isolated guinea-pig left auricle. J. Pharmacol., **145**, 162.

21 Harigaya, S. and Schwartz, A. (1969). Rate of calcium binding and uptake in normal animal and failing human cardiac muscle. Circ. Res., **25**, 781.

22 Hartshorne, D.J. and Mueller, H. (1967). Separation and recombination of the ethylene glycol bis(β-aminoethyl ether)-N, N'-tetraacetic acid-sensitizing factor obtained from a low ionic strength extract of natural actomyosin. J. biol. Chem., **242**, 3089.

23 Hartshorne, D.J., Theiner, M. and Mueller, H. (1969). Studies on troponin. Biochim. biophys. acta, **175**, 301.

24 Hartshorne, D.J. (1970). Interactions of desensitized actomyosin with tropomyosin, troponin A, troponin B and polyanions. J. gen. Physiol., **55**, 585.

25 Hasselbach, W. and Makinose, M. (1961). Die Calciumpumpe der "Erschlaffungsrana" des Muskels und ihre Abhängigkeit von der ATP-Spaltung. Biochem. Z., **333**, 518.

26 Heilbrun, L.V. and Wiercinski, F.J. (1947). The action of various cations in muscle protoplasm. J. cell. comp. Physiol., **29**, 15.

27 Huxley, A.F. and Niedergierke, R. (1954). Structural changes in muscle during contraction. Interference microscopy of living muscle fibres. Nature, Lond., **173**, 971.

28 Huxley, H.E. and Hansen, J. (1954). Changes in the cross striations of muscle during contraction and stretch, and their structural interpretation. Nature, Lond., **173**, 973.

29 Huxley, H.E. (1969). The mechanism of muscular contraction. Science, **164**, 1356.

30 Katz, A. and Repke, D.I. (1967). Quantitative aspects of dog cardiac microsomal binding and calcium uptake. Circ. Res., **21**, 153.

31 Kielley, W.W. and Meyerhof, O. (1948). A new magnesium activated adenosine-triphosphatase from muscle. J. biol. Chem., **174**, 387.

32 Kübler, W. and Shinebourne, E.A. (This symposium.)

33 Kumagai, H., Ebashi, S. and Takeda, F. (1955). Essential relaxing factor in muscle other than myokinase and creatine phosphokinase. Nature, Lond., **176**, 166.

34 Lain, R.F., Hess, M.L., Gertz, E.W. and Briggs, F.N. (1968). Calcium uptake activity of canine myocardial sarcoplasmic reticulum in the presence of anesthetic agents. Circ.Res., **23**, 597.

35 Langer, G.A. (1965). Calcium exchange in dog ventricular muscle: Relation to frequency of contraction and maintenance of contractility. Circ.Res., **17**, 78.

36 Lee, K.S., Ladinsky, H. and Stuckey, J.H. (1967). Decreased Ca^{++} uptake by sarcoplasmic reticulum after coronary artery occlusion for 60 and 90 minutes. Circ. Res., **21**, 439.

37 Lee, K.S. and Choi, S.J. (1966). Effects of the cardiac glycosides on the Ca^{++} uptake of cardiac sarcoplasmic reticulum. J.Pharmacol., **153**, 114.

38 Locke, F.S. and Rosenheim, O. (1907). Contributions to the physiology of the isolated heart. The consumption of dextrose by mammalian cardiac muscle. J.Physiol., **36**, 205.

39 Lowey, S., Slayter, H.S., Weeds, A.G. and Baker, H. (1969). Substructure of the myosin molecule. I. Subfragments of myosin by enzymic degradation. J.molec.Biol., **42**, 1.

40 Marsh, B.B. (1951). A factor modifying muscle fiber syneresis. Nature, Lond., **167**, 1065.

41 Morales, M.F., Botts, J., Blum, J.J. and Hill, T.L. (1955). Elementary processes in muscle action: An examination of current concepts. Physiol.Rev., **35**, 474.

42 Mueller, H., Franzen, J., Rice, R.V. and Olson, R.E. (1964). Characterization of cardiac myosin from the dog. J.biol.Chem., **239**, 1447.

43 Muir, J.R., Dhalla, N.S., Orteza, J.M. and Olson, R.E. (1970). Energy-linked calcium transport in subcellular fractions of the failing rat heart. Circ.Res., **26**, 429.

44 Muir, J.R., Weber, A. and Olson, R.E. (1970). Properties of cardiac myofibrillar ATP-ase. Biochim.biophys. acta (in press).

45 Nayler, W.G. (1960). A study of the "staircase" in ventricular muscle and its relationship to the inotropic activity of certain drugs. J. gen. Physiol., **44**, 393.

46 Niedergierke, R. (1963). Movements of calcium in frog heart ventricles at rest and during contractures. J. Physiol., **167**, 551.

47 Olson, R.E. and Schwartz, W.B. (1951). Myocardiac metabolism in congestive heart failure. Medicine, **30**, 21.

48 Patriarca, P. and Carafoli, E. (1968). A study of the intracellular transport of calcium in rat heart. J. cell. comp. Physiol., **72**, 29.

49 Perry, S.V. and Grey, T.C. (1956). A study of the effects of substrate concentration and certain relaxing factors on the magnesium-activated myofibrillar adenosine triphosphatase. Biochem. J., **64**, 184.

50 Perry, S.V. and Grey, T.C. (1958). Ethylenediaminetetraacetic acid and the adenosinetriphosphatase activity of actomyosin systems. Biochem. J., **64**, 58.

51 Ringer, S. (1882). A further contribution regarding the influence of the different constituents of the blood on the contraction of the heart. J. Physiol., **4**, 29.

52 Watanabe, S. (1955). Relaxing effects of EDTA on glycerol treated muscle fibers. Arch. Biochem. Biophys., **54**, 559.

53 Weber, A. (1959). On the role of calcium in the activity of adenosine-5'-triphosphate hydrolysis by actomyosin. J. biol. Chem., **234**, 2764.

54 Weber, A. and Winicur, S. (1961). The rôle of calcium in the superprecipitation of actomyosin. J. biol. Chem., **236**, 3198.

55 Weber, A., Herz, R. and Reiss, I. (1967). The nature of the cardiac relaxing factor. Biochim. biophys. acta, **131**, 188.

56 Weber, H.H. (1934). The muscle proteins and the finer structure of skeletal muscles. Ergebn. Physiol., **36**, 109.

57 Winegrad, S. and Shanes, A.M. (1962). Calcium flux and contractility of guinea pig atria. J. gen. Physiol., **45**, 371.

CELLULAR EXCHANGE OF CALCIUM*

WINIFRED G. NAYLER AND N.C.R. MERRILLEES

Baker Medical Research Institute, Melbourne, Australia
and
Department of Anatomy, University of Melbourne,
Parkville, Victoria, Australia

I. INTRODUCTION

It is now generally agreed that contraction in striated muscle involves an interaction between the myofibrillar proteins, actin and myosin.[27, 28, 30, 37, 60, 84, 95] This reaction is triggered by ionized calcium (Ca^{2+}) and energy for it is derived from adenosine triphosphate.[7, 11, 70] The intracellular Ca^{2+} concentration determines the rate of adenosine triphosphate splitting, and hence the rate of tension development.[30, 93, 95] Reconstituted actomysin, prepared from purified actin and myosin, fails to contract in the presence of ATP and Ca^{2+} unless two other proteins are

---

*This investigation was supported by grants-in-aid from the National Heart Foundation of Australia and the Life Insurance Medical Research Fund of Australia and New Zealand.

added.[13, 19, 24] These proteins, troponin and tropomyosin, are both normally present in striated muscle and apparently form a complex which sensitizes actomyosin to Ca^{2+}. When Ca^{2+} is either absent or its concentration falls below a critical level, the troponin-tropomyosin complex inhibits the interaction between actin and myosin and the associated activation of the actomyosin ATPase enzyme. When the Ca^{2+} concentration exceeds a critical level the inhibitory effect of the troponin-tropomyosin complex is abolished, and the interaction between actin and myosin and the associated activation of the ATPase enzyme can occur.[13, 19] These events are shown schematically in Fig. 1. The Ca^{2+} required to activate this system ranges between 10^{-5} M and 10^{-7} M,[95] a range which is of the same order as that required for the activation of contraction in intact muscle fibres.[69, 72] The Ca^{2+}-binding activity of the troponin-tropomyosin complex resides in the troponin moiety.[13]

II. DISTRIBUTION OF Ca^{2+} IN CARDIAC MUSCLE

Cardiac muscle contains approximately 2.5 mM Ca^{2+} per litre tissue water,[12] a concentration far in excess of the activation threshold concentration of 5×10^{-7} M.[72] Despite the presence of this relatively high concentration of Ca^{2+}, excitation of cardiac muscle which is immersed in a Ca^{2+}-free solution[79] fails to elicit a mechanical response, although the action potential itself persists.[41, 46] If it is agreed that the intracellular concentration of Ca^{2+} is the major determinant of the speed and magnitude of contraction in cardiac muscle, and that during diastole (or

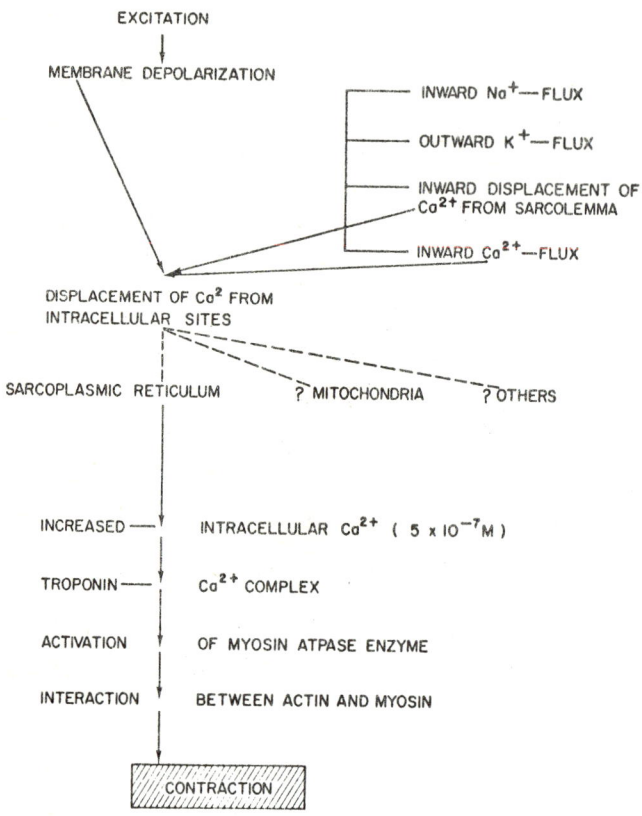

Fig. 1. Schematic representation of excitation-contraction coupling in heart muscle.

relaxation) the intracellular concentration of Ca^{2+} falls below the activation threshold concentration, then it follows that it is only when the extracellular phase contains Ca^{2+} that excitation causes the intracellular concentration of Ca^{2+} to exceed the activation threshold level. Theoretically Ca^{2+} from the extracellular phase could be involved directly. Alternatively initiation of the mechanical response may depend upon the release of Ca^{2+} from cellular stores which are maintained only if the extracellular phase contains Ca^{2+}; or the presence of Ca^{2+} in the extracellular phase may facilitate an excitation-induced displacement of Ca^{2+} from cellular storage depots.

Studies relating to the intracellular distribution of Ca^{2+} in muscle cells have shown it to occur in association with many subcellular structures, including the myofibrils, mitochondria, nuclei, myoplasm, sarcolemma and sarcoplasmic reticulum (see ref. 50 for bibliography). Presumably, Ca^{2+} which is stored in these subcellular structures is bound to them in such a way that, in the absence of extracellular Ca^{2+}, it is not available for excitation-contraction-coupling,[83, 84] even when the plasma membrane is fully depolarized,[59] unless drugs which displace Ca^{2+} from cellular binding sites are introduced.[35, 49, 51]

Radioisotope studies have confirmed that the distribution of Ca^{2+} in cardiac muscle is complex and compartmentalized. Winegrad and Shanes[100] found kinetic evidence for three components of Ca^{2+}-exchange in guinea pig atria: rapidly-exchangeable, slowly-exchangeable and non-exchangeable. These made up 59%, 15% and 26% respectively of atrial Ca^{2+}. The half-life of the rapidly-exchangeable fraction (4.5 min) is too long for it to be accounted for in terms of the extracellular phase and suggests an accumulation of Ca^{2+} at a site intermediate between extra- and intracellular phases. In arterially-perfused, isolated dog papillary muscles, Langer and Brady[38] detected at least five phases of Ca^{2+} exchange, one with a half-life of only 6.0 minutes. Several phases of Ca^{2+} exchange have been described for rabbit ventricular muscle[86] and again the half-life of one of these phases is too short for it to be accounted for in terms of the extracellular space, yet too long for it to be derived from an intracellular site. The organelles which act as cellular depots for this rapidly-exchangeable and, therefore, presumably superficially-located Ca^{2+}-fraction have not been positively identified. Possibly they include:—

(a) **The sarcolemma.** There is complete cell separation at the intercalated disc. The plasma membranes of two apposed cells are separated by a narrow extracellular space which is continuous with the general extracellular space. Although the relationships of the membranes are modified in places by small areas of gap-junction, these evidently do not interfere with the free communication between the general and the intercalated-disc extracellular spaces. Colloidal lanthanum hydroxide[78] penetrates freely into the spaces of the gap (Fig. 2). Ionic exchange between the intra- and extracellular phases, therefore, may take place at the intercalated disc as at the remainder of the sarcolemma, including its ramifications as the transverse tubular system (T system).

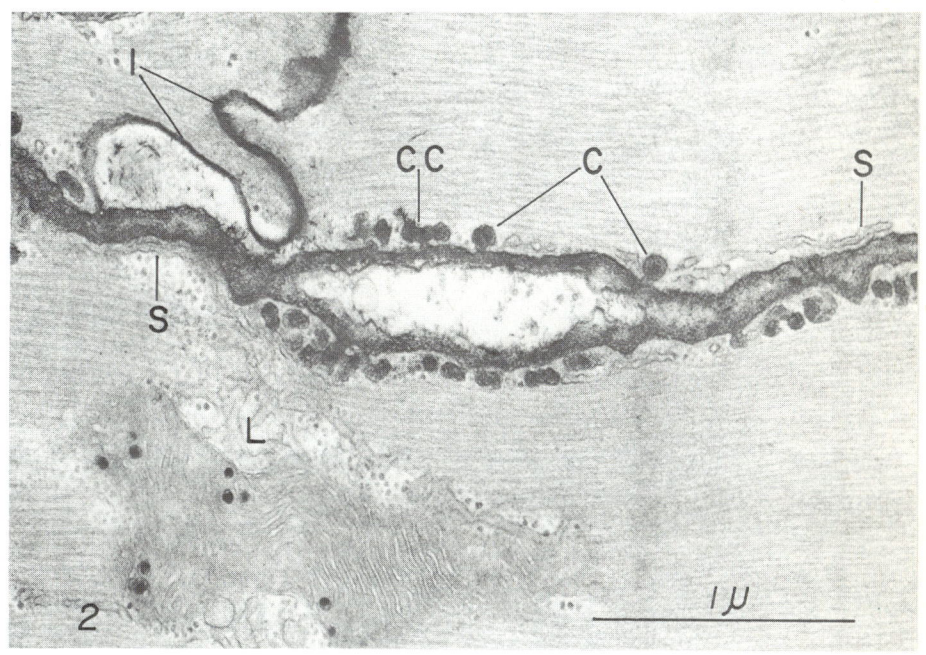

Fig. 2. Dog papillary muscle processed with lanthanum hydroxide. The dense material has filled the intercellular spaces including gap-junction and close-contact zones of an intercalated disc (I), and has filled the 'caveolae intracellulares' (C), some of which are complex (CC). The hydroxide has not entered the longitudinal sarcoplasmic reticulum (L) or its extensions, the subsarcolemmal cisternae (S), which have no connection with the extracellular space. The size and density of the mitochondrial granules are not related to the lanthanum hydroxide treatment.

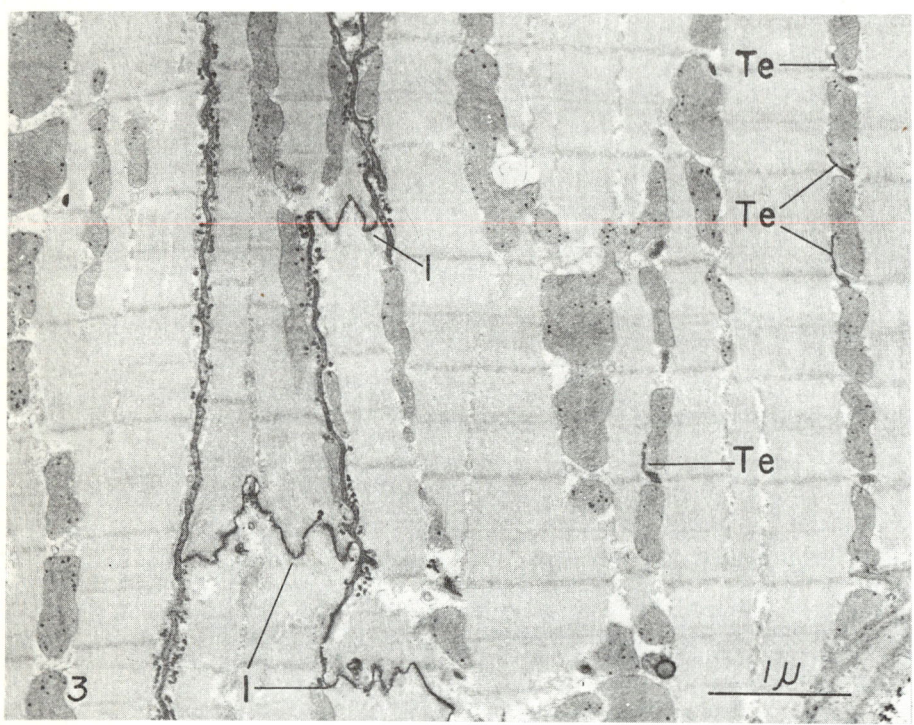

Fig. 3. Dog papillary muscle processed with colloidal lanthanum hydroxide. The extracellular spaces, including those in intercalated discs (I), 'caveolae intracellulares' or micropinocytotic vesicles, and transverse tubules are filled with dense deposit. The field includes an unusually large proportion of transverse tubules with longitudinally-directed, thin extensions (Te).

(b) **The transverse tubular system.** The transverse tubular system consists of a ramifying network of tubules of various diameters continuous with the sarcolemma and open to the extracellular space.[56, 73, 88, 89] The transverse tubule system is generally confined to the plane of the Z band, but longitudinally-directed branches are common. Forssmann and Girardier[18] described a range of sizes of branches in the rat heart, the larger being of the same general diameter as the rest of the system. Figs. 3 and 4 show that the thin longitudinally-running branches of the T system reported by Forssmann and Girardier[18] for rat ventricle also occur in the dog. Although the possible involvement of the transverse tubular system in excitation-contraction-coupling in mammalian heart muscle is well documented,[37] whether or not Ca^{2+} is stored in this system (or its ramifications) for subsequent release remains to be demonstrated.[65]

(c) **The longitudinal elements of the sarcoplasmic reticulum and its associated cisternae.** (See refs. 4, 17, 71 for bibliography.) As shown by the electron micrograph in Fig. 2, this system consists of a ramifying network of tubules which are separated from the extracellular space and therefore contain no colloidal lanthanum hydroxide. In contrast with the arrangement found in skeletal muscle, where the longitudinal reticulum is not continuous across sarcomere boundaries along the myofibrils, in cardiac muscle the system is continuous through the muscle cell. Special branches of the system become modified whenever they form a close contact with the sarcolemma and its invaginations. The

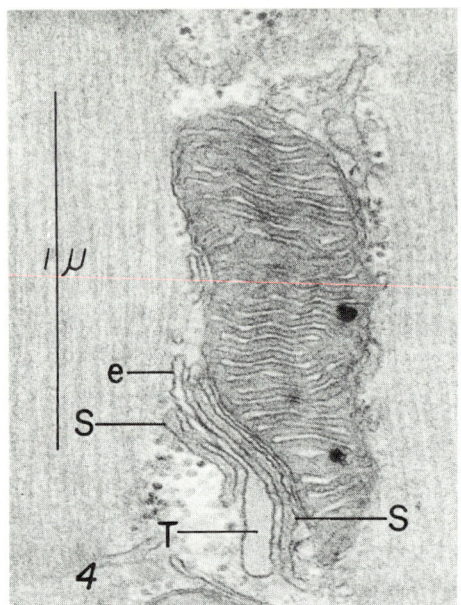

Fig. 4. Dog papillary muscle. Two subsarcolemmal cisternae (S) lie along the transverse tubule (T) and its longitudinally-directed thin extension (e). The material in the extension is less dense than that in the subsarcolemmal cisternae, which are continuous with the longitudinal system of the sarcoplasmic reticulum.

special branches are the sub-sarcolemmal cisternae[81] and their appearance is constant irrespective of whether they are under the sarcolemma or along the T tubule system and also regardless of the orientation or diameter of the T tubule[90] (Fig. 4). The distance that separates the sub-sarcolemmal cisternae and, therefore, the longitudinal reticulum system, from the extracellular space is small.

It is generally believed that Ca^{2+} is stored in the cisternae of the longitudinal reticulum and that during excitation-contraction coupling Ca^{2+} is released as the result of activity at the T-tubule-reticulum junction.[9, 16, 25, 67, 68]

(d) **The Z tubules.** In some mammalian heart muscle a system of tubules known as the Z tubules[88, 90] encircle the bundles of myofilaments at the level of the Z band. These tubules are absent from cat heart muscle.[17] The Z tubules are approximately 200 to 400 Å in diameter and neighbouring tubules communicate with one another in such a way that they are linked across the cell, closely applied to the Z band. Evidence of these tubules is clearly shown in the electron micrograph reproduced in Fig. 5, which is a longitudinal section of perfusion-fixed dog heart muscle. These Z tubules are a transversely oriented part of the longitudinal reticulum.[90]

(e) **Mitochondria.** Lastly, another source of rapidly-exchangeable Ca^{2+} may be the mitochondria. Forssmann and Girardier[18] noted the close association between mitochondria and T tubules in cardiac muscle.

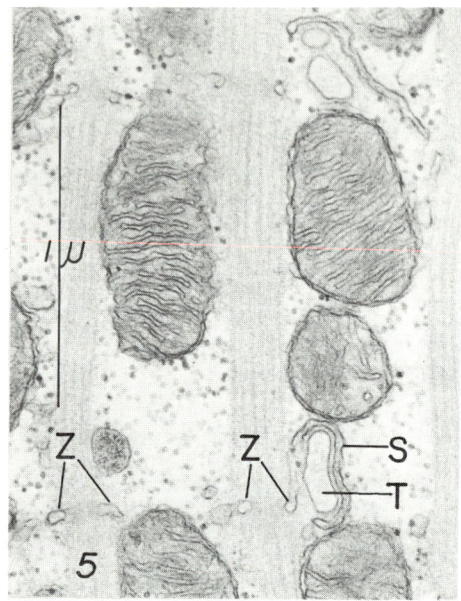

Fig. 5. Dog papillary muscle. The transverse tubule (T), containing basement membrane material, is separated from the subsarcolemmal cisternae (S) by a gap of less than 200 Å. Profiles of the transversely-running, Z-tubule component (Z) of the longitudinal reticulum are conspicuous in the dog, and most of the subsarcolemmal cisternae appear to arise from that component.

III. CALCIUM EXCHANGE ASSOCIATED WITH THE ACTION POTENTIAL

Provided that the extracellular phase contains Ca^{2+}, reduction of the transmembrane resting potential below a critical level (approximately -50 mV) elicits contraction in heart muscle. At the same time the permeability of the cell membrane to Ca^{2+} is increased.[10, 76] Using a voltage clamp technique to study inward currents associated with the **rapid phase** of depolarization of the action potential,[26] Beeler and Reuter[3] demonstrated that, in addition to the large **rapid** inward Na^+ current that is predominant during phase 0 of the action potential and is shown schematically in Fig. 6, there is a relatively **slow** inward current, the existence of which depends upon Ca^{2+} being present in the extracellular phase. This slow inward current is a Ca^{2+} current,[2, 3] the charge carrier for which is Ca^{2+}. In cardiac muscle the rapid inward Na^+ current is probably responsible for depolarizing the membrane to a level at which the inward Ca^{2+} current is readily activated.[2, 3, 45]

Evidence that Ca^{2+} contribute current during the **plateau phase** of the action potential was provided by the earlier experiments of Reuter.[74, 75] Many other investigations, including those of Niedergerke and Orkand,[63] substantiate the hypothesis that the **inward current during the action potential is carried by Ca^{2+} as well as Na^+**. Possibly, as Niedergerke and Orkand[63] suggested, the effect of the inward Ca^{2+} current is negligible during the initial fast upstroke phase of the action potential (phase 0 in Fig.

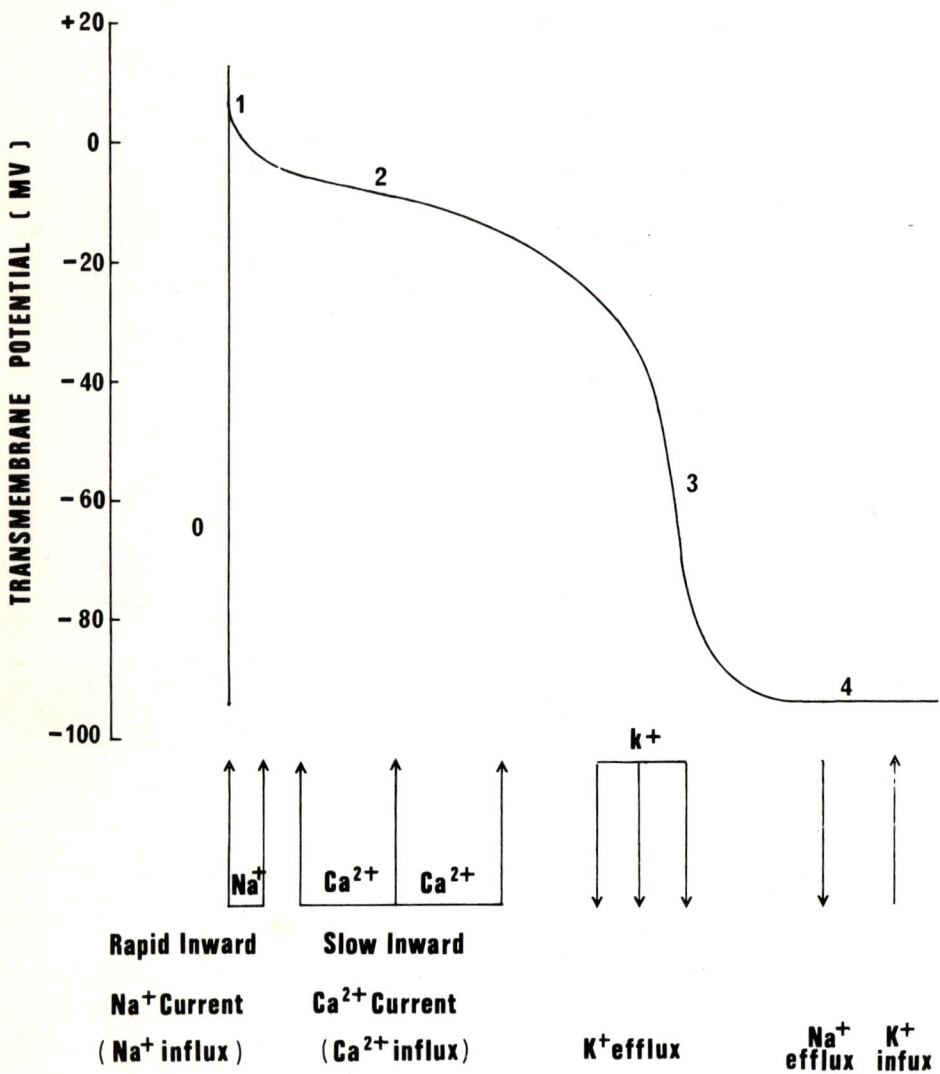

Fig. 6. Schematic representation of ion fluxes associated with an action potential in heart muscle.

6), when the current is carried mainly by Na^+. During the late part of the rising phase of the action potential, however, when the permeability to Na^+ and K^+ is declining, the inward Ca^{2+} current may be a significant factor in contributing to the height and maintenance of the plateau potential.

If this slow inward current reflects an excitation-induced inward-displacement of Ca^{2+}, then the question arises as to whether or not the Ca^{2+} involved is sufficient to raise the myoplasmic concentration of Ca^{2+} above the activation threshold for contraction.

Guinea pig atria, which are immersed in a Ca^{45}-labelled physiological saline solution containing 2.5 mM Ca^{2+} and stimulated to contract at a rate of 30 beats per minute, accumulate 0.55 μμmole $^{45}Ca^{2+}$ per cm^2 per beat in excess of the resting influx (0.029 μμmole per cm^2 per second.[100] Data from Winegrad and Shanes' experiments,[100] summarized in Fig. 7, show that the magnitude of this 'extra' Ca^{2+} influx is influenced (a) by the extracellular Ca^{2+} concentration, and (b) by the frequency with which contraction occurs. These findings have been confirmed and extended for heart muscle from a variety of species.[22,35,51,61] In general the 'extra' Ca^{2+} influx associated with each action potential ranges between 0.5 and 2.7 μmole per kg per beat, depending upon the species, the frequency with which stimulation occurs and the extracellular Ca^{2+} and Na^+ concentration. Generally, however, the additional influx is matched by an extra efflux and, therefore, there is no overall but only a momentary gain in Ca^{2+}. Dog papillary muscle provides an exception to this rule:

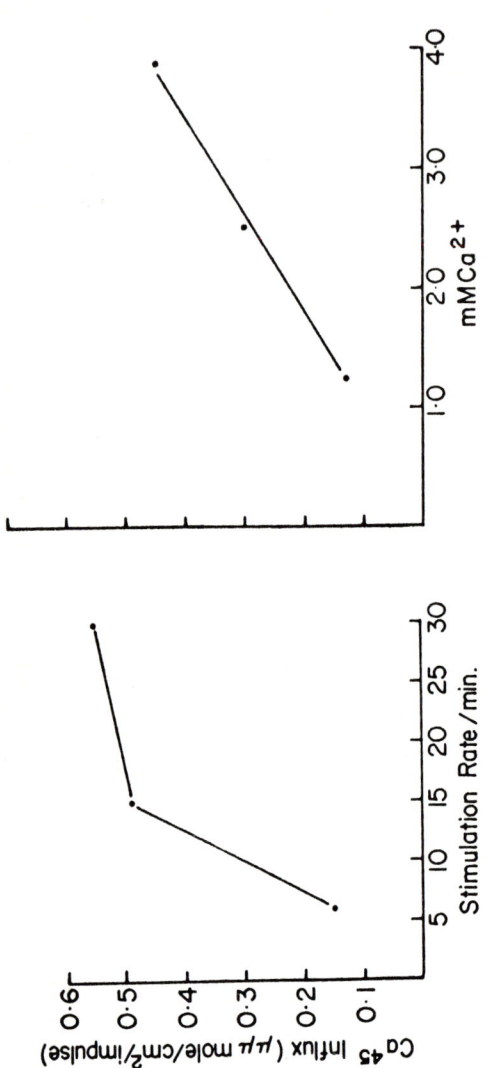

Fig. 7. Effect of stimulation rate and of extracellular Ca^{2+} on the uptake of Ca^{2+} (detected as $^{45}Ca^{2+}$) by isolated guinea pig atria. (Data from Winegrad and Shanes.[100])

Langer and Brady[38] found that an increase of 27 stimuli per minute in the rate with which excitation was induced resulted in an average increase in Ca^{2+} influx of 1.9 μmole per kg per beat. Dog heart muscle is peculiar in that Ca^{2+} efflux lags behind Ca^{2+} influx and Langer and Brady[38] detected a net increment of 0.5 m.mole Ca^{2+} per kg heart weight after 10 minutes' stimulation at a rate of 27 per minute in excess of that used previously. The Ca^{2+} responsible for this gain, like that associated with a reduction in extracellular Na^+,[35] is localized in that portion of the muscle defined kinetically as phase 2, i.e. it is the rapidly-exchangeable fraction. It has been calculated[94, 31] that 50 μ moles Ca^{2+} per kg wet weight is sufficient to saturate the actomyosin of mammalian heart muscle, with respect to full activation of the actomyosin ATPase enzyme. In dog papillary muscle, therefore, if all the increment of Ca^{2+} influx (0.5 m.mole per kg) were transferred directly to the contractile proteins **with each** beat, then the actomyosin ATPase enzyme should be fully activated. In heart muscle in general, however, the 'extra' Ca^{2+} influx associated with each excitation apparently is insufficient to account for activation of this ATPase enzyme and, therefore, is probably insufficient by itself to activate the process of contraction.

This argument may be inconclusive, however, because if a large Ca^{2+} influx during depolarization is followed by an equally large efflux during repolarization, then the currently used techniques for measuring Ca^{2+} influx may yield erroneously low results, because they do not allow for the complete separation of efflux from influx.

IV. CALCIUM EXCHANGE AND THE ACTIVATION OF CONTRACTION

There is ample evidence that Ca^{2+} facilitates contraction in heart muscle, that heart muscle accumulates Ca^{2+} under conditions of increased contractility[36, 37, 39, 51, 59, 62, 64, 79, 82, 98] and that the link between the action potential and the activation of the mechanical response depends upon the presence of Ca^{2+} in the extracellular phase. The 'extra' Ca^{2+} influx associated with each action potential, although insufficient by itself to activate contraction, probably provides the basis for the well documented relationship which exists between the tension developed during contraction and the frequency with which contraction occurs (the 'staircase' phenomenon) and post-stimulation potentiation.[33, 36, 51, 57, 80, 98] Thus, unless this additional Ca^{2+} is all rapidly sequestered and bound at intracellular binding sites, it must result in a raised intracellular Ca^{2+} concentration. Similarly the 'extra' Ca^{2+} influx associated with a raised extracellular Ca^{2+} (Fig. 7) probably contributes to the mechanism whereby the developed tension is proportional to the extracellular Ca^{2+}.[61]

The effect on contraction of a changed extracellular Ca^{2+} concentration develops rapidly.[59] The sites at which the Ca^{2+} exert their effect, therefore, must be in close proximity to the extracellular space, i.e. they must be superficially-located sites.[61] Possibly, there is a rapid, direct exchange of Ca^{2+} across the cell membrane, and hence a rapid, direct exchange of Ca^{2+} between the extra- and intracellular phases. Alternatively, the Ca^{2+} exchange involved may not reflect a direct exchange of Ca^{2+} between intra- and extracellular phases but instead the displacement of Ca^{2+} from superficially-located binding sites in the immediate vicinity of, or within, the cell membrane itself. Theoretically, during relaxation, Ca^{2+} stored in these superficially-located depots may be in equilibrium with the extracellular Ca^{2+}, and during excitation may be displaced into the myoplasm where it can activate contraction either directly or indirectly, by displacing additional Ca^{2+} from other intracellular storage depots, shown schematically in Fig. 8.

Niedergerke's tracer experiments[59] showed that in frog heart muscle the amount of Ca^{2+} involved in the contractile response is at least four times greater than that found in the extracellular phase, indicating that in frog heart muscle, changes in contractile tension due to an altered extracellular Ca^{2+} concentration necessarily involve an initial cellular accumulation of Ca^{2+}. The rapid time-course of the response indicates that this accumulation takes place at superficially-located loci. This conclusion is supported by the fact that although the time-course of the tension change which results from an altered extracellular Ca^{2+} can be fitted to an equation describing the diffusion of Ca^{2+} through the interstitial space, the 'apparent' diffusion coefficient for Ca^{2+} is only one fourth of that expected for diffusion through the extracellular space.[59]

In considering possible membrane-located sites at which Ca^{2+} binding or accumulation might occur, it can be argued that since toad and frog heart muscle respond rapidly to a changed

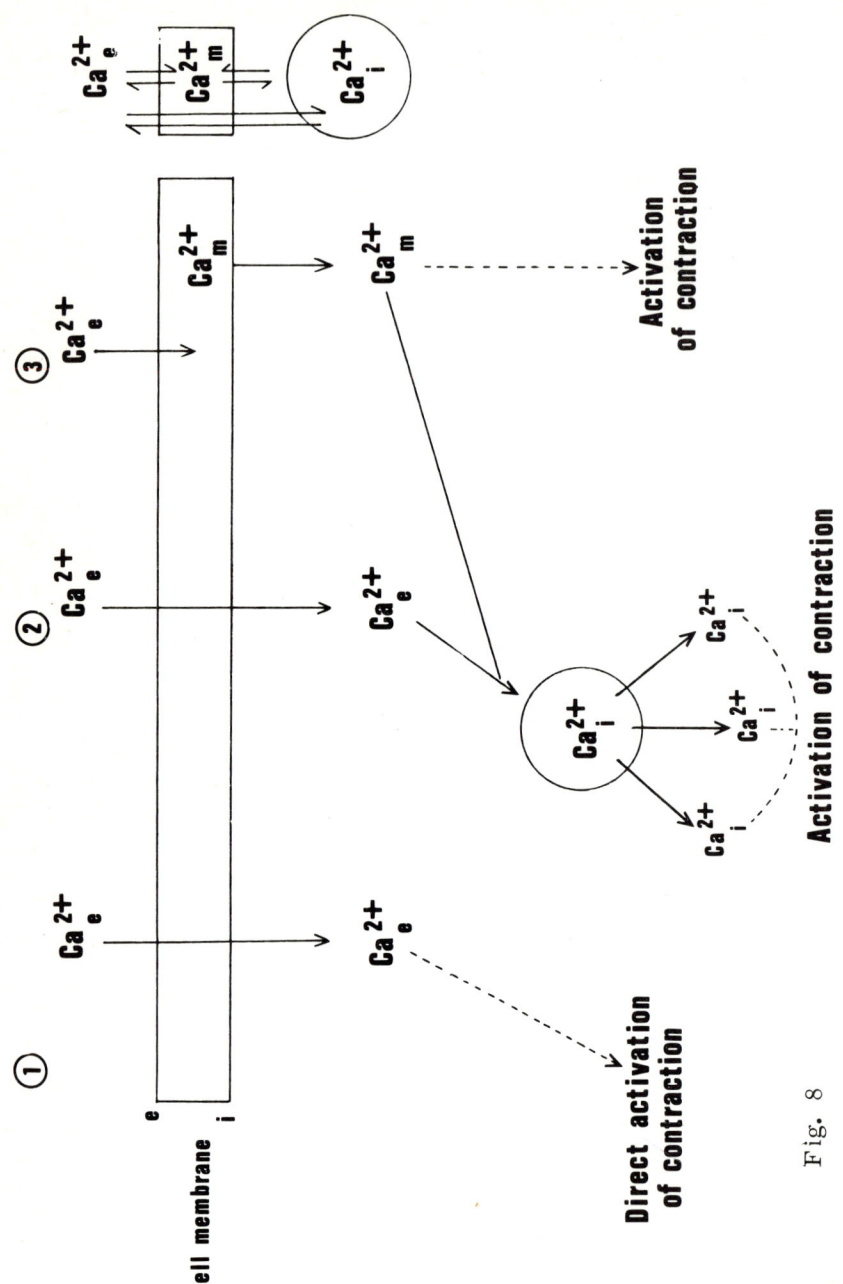

Fig. 8

extracellular concentration of Ca^{2+} despite the absence of a T system$^{53,\ 91}$ the response cannot depend upon the accumulation of Ca^{2+} in a T system. Theoretically Ca^{2+} could accumulate at superficially-located sites on the cell membrane and be transported into the myoplasm by pinocytosis, the amount of Ca^{2+} stored at the superficially-located sites being determined by the extracellular $(Ca^{2+})/(Na^+)^2$ ratio.$^{43,\ 97}$ It is generally believed, however, that the rate at which the micropinocytotic vesicles form is too slow for this process to be responsible for a rapid change in the intracellular Ca^{2+} concentration. It has been argued that the small size of cardiac muscle cells^{56} makes unnecessary the development of specialized structures ensuring the rapid inward spread of excitation, and that the simple diffusion of an exchangeable but previously bound fraction of Ca^{2+} (activator Ca^{2+}) from the excited plasma membrane to the contractile proteins would be fast enough to permit synchronization of contraction. Probably this is true for amphibian heart muscle, where contraction is slow compared with that found, for example, in rat or dog heart muscle.

This argument, that simple diffusion can account for the inward spread of the Ca^{2+} which will activate contraction, is based on the assumption that the rate at which Ca^{2+} diffuses from the plasma membrane through the myoplasm to the myofibrils is the

---

Fig. 8. Schematic representation of Ca^{2+} exchange across the cell membrane during excitation.
Ca_e^{2+} refers to Ca^{2+} from the extracellular phase, Ca_m^{2+} to membrane-located Ca^{2+}, and Ca_i^{2+} to Ca^{2+} from the intracellular phase.

same as that which applies to the diffusion of Ca^{2+} in aqueous solutions. Because the myoplasm contains many organelles, some of which are capable of sequestering Ca^{2+}, the rate at which Ca^{2+} diffuses through the myoplasm may be significantly different from that found in aqueous solutions. Specialized pathways therefore may be needed to direct the activator-Ca^{2+} to the immediate vicinity of the contractile proteins.

Müller's experiments[48] could be interpreted as providing evidence in support of this latter hypothesis. Using dog and sheep trabecular muscle, Müller found that cardiac muscle does not respond to local stimulation by local contraction as does skeletal muscle.[27, 29] Instead the contraction spreads over several sarcomeres. One interpretation of Müller's results is that the spread of excitation reflects the fact that the longitudinal reticulum of cardiac muscle is continuous throughout the length of each cell and, as already stated, is not interrupted between sarcomeres as it is in skeletal muscle. An alternative explanation is that sub-threshold depolarization in mammalian heart muscle activates the release of Ca^{2+} from storage sites immediately below the sarcolemma, possibly from the sub-sarcolemmal cisternae[65, 81] of the longitudinal reticulum. Diffusion through the lumen of the T tubules of previously bound ions made exchangeable as the result of membrane depolarization is probably compartmentalized and restricted, even though the lumen of the T tubule in mammalian heart muscle is in direct communication with the extracellular space.[89] The T system is tortuous and the diameter of its lumen varies over a wide range (between 1000 and

300 Å in rat ventricular muscle). However, because of the areas of close contact between the longitudinal components of the sarcoplasmic reticulum and the transverse tubular system, Fahrenbach's suggestion[16] that the effect of membrane depolarization extends directly to the longitudinal reticulum and its specialized regions is generally accepted.

Microsomal vesicles prepared from heart muscle by the currently used methods of homogenization, differential centrifugation and sucrose gradient purification probably contain fragments of membranes which, in intact muscle cells, are essentially associated with the sarcolemma, the T tubules and the longitudinal components of the sarcoplasmic reticulum. Biochemical studies have repeatedly shown that these microsomal vesicles can accumulate and bind Ca^{2+} against large concentration gradients,[31,44] that Ca^{2+} and Na^+ compete for microsomal binding sites,[66] and that Ca^{2+} can be displaced from the vesicles by a variety of stimuli, including that of electrical stimulation.[40,85] If it is assumed that the sarcolemma and its specialized regions (the intercalated disc and the T tubules) and the longitudinal reticulum and its specialized regions (the sub-sarcolemmal cisternae and the Z tubules) respond to excitation, then it can be argued that the Ca^{2+} stored in this system under in-vivo conditions corresponds to the rapidly exchangeable, superficially-located fraction of Ca^{2+}, defined kinetically as phase 2 by Langer and Brady.[38] In this case this represents the site at which Ca^{2+} accumulates in response to either an increase in the frequency with which contraction is initiated or a raised extracellular Ca^{2+}.

V. MEMBRANE DEPOLARIZATION AND THE ACTIVATION OF CONTRACTION

The precise mechanism whereby membrane depolarization triggers a release of previously bound Ca^{2+}, and hence increases the concentration of exchangeable Ca^{2+} in the myoplasm, is obscure. The failure of short periods of depolarization (1-5 m. sec) to produce substantial or even detectable tension[47] indicates that a minimum period of depolarization is required. The level of depolarization influences the developed tension[47] and the development of tension is facilitated if the membrane potential is maintained at a positive level. The most rapid rate of tension development occurs during the early rising phase of the action potential; this may simply reflect the time during the action potential when the membrane potential is positive. Because tension development can proceed **after** the membrane has been repolarized to its resting state[47] it seems probable that the contractile process persists for a period of time once it has been activated. The relative rate of tension development during the early stages of the action potential is known to be a function of the extracellular Ca^{2+}, and artificially lengthening the action potential alters the time course and amplitude of the contraction only within the early stages of the action potential. These findings and others[2, 3, 32, 96, 101] support the hypothesis that in cardiac muscle the action potential not only acts as a trigger but also as the determinant of the duration and, to some extent, the magnitude of the mechanical response.

During the onset of the mechanical response the main increase in the force of contraction develops in the potential range when the inward driving force for Na^+ is small and that for Ca^{2+} is large (see Fig. 6). The principal tension development can be exclusively correlated to this Ca^{2+} influx.[3, 101] Moreover, provided that the extracellular phase contains Na^+, **the development of tension is preceded by and does not occur simultaneously with the Ca^{2+} influx.** Under these conditions changes in the duration of the action potential in mammalian cardiac muscle do not have instantaneous effects on the tension developed.[101, 1] Instead several cycles of depolarization are needed to establish a new steady state with respect to the action potential and developed tension.

Possibly, when the extracellular phase contains Na^+, those Ca^{2+} which flow into the cell during depolarization are either rapidly inactivated or sequestered, before any activation of contraction occurs, and the Ca^{2+} which activates contraction is displaced from intracellular binding sites by a mechanism dependent upon depolarization. The amount of Ca^{2+} stored at these intracellular sites would depend upon a balance between the extracellular $Ca^{2+}/(Na^+)^2$, the charge transfer carried by Ca^{2+} during preceding depolarizations, and the rate at which Ca^{2+} is extruded from the intra- to the extracellular phase. Ca^{2+} efflux is dependent upon the presence of Na^+ in the extracellular phase.[77, 6] In the absence of Na^+, Ca^{2+} efflux is inhibited and there is a large cellular uptake of Ca^{2+} which[35] is localized in the rapidly-exchangeable fraction defined kinetically as phase 2. Under these conditions an increasing number of membrane-located binding sites are already occupied by Ca^{2+}, before depolarization occurs. In Na^+-free solutions, twitch tension appears to be **directly** related to the inward Ca^{2+} current, and repetitive depolarization results in contracture,[23] a result which would be anticipated if all the binding sites for Ca^{2+} were fully occupied before depolarization occurred, so that none of the Ca^{2+} associated with the inward Ca^{2+} current of the action potential need be bound and inactivated.

The increased strength of contraction which results from a reduction in the interval between beats can, as already explained, be accounted for in terms of the enhanced Ca^{2+} influx which occurs under these conditions. If, however, a period of relatively rapid excitation is followed by a pause then, as shown in the tracing in the first panel of Fig. 10, the first beat after the pause is potentiated.

A rational explanation for this 'post-stimulation potentiation'[80] is found in the suggestion that the Ca^{2+} which is made available to the myofibrils for the activation of contraction originates from at least two sources, one of which involves the Ca^{2+} influx associated with the initial depolarization, and the other Ca^{2+} which can be displaced from cellular storage sites as the result of membrane depolarization.

If it is agreed that the amount of Ca^{2+} stored at these cellular sites is determined by the myoplasmic Ca^{2+} concentration achieved during the previous series of events,[101] and that time is required either for the binding or the translocation of Ca^{2+} to specific sites from which it can be released during subsequent depolarization,

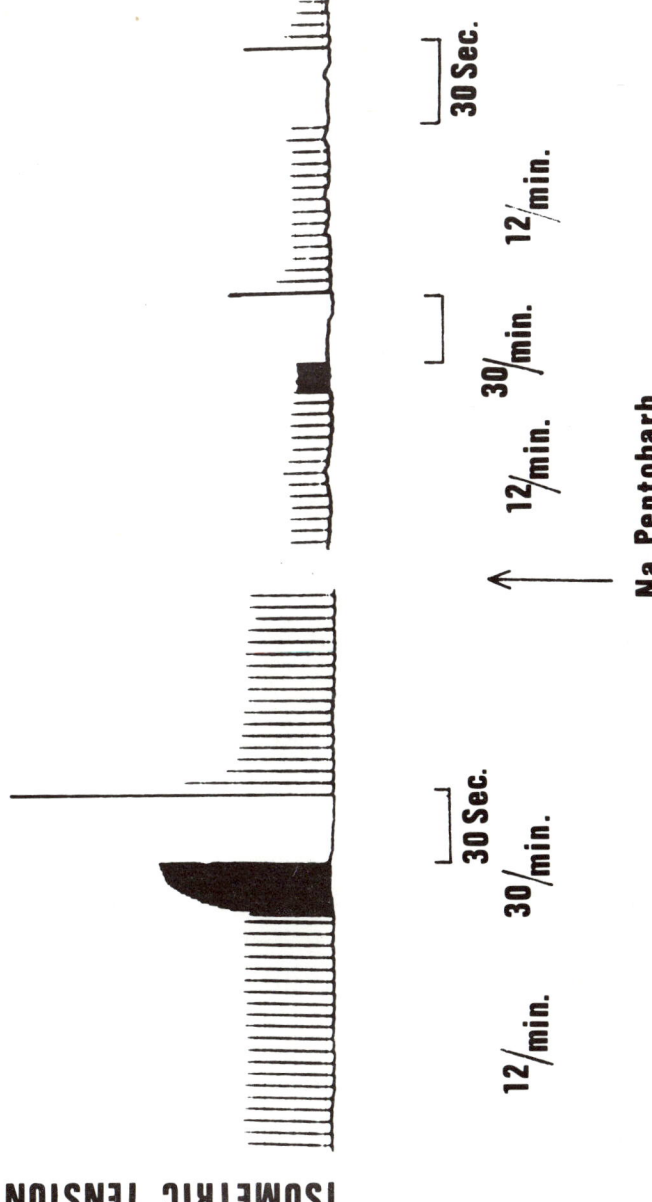

Fig. 9. Isometric tension recorded from isolated dog trabecular muscle immersed in Tyrode's solution at 35° C and stimulated to contract at the indicated rates. Rest intervals (30 seconds) were applied as shown. At arrow, sodium pentobarbitone was added to provide a final concentration of 100 μM.

then the fact that the first twitch following a pause after a period of rapid excitations is potentiated, as shown in Fig. 9, can be explained. Presumably the fraction of Ca^{2+} which is accumulated and then released is located within the various ramifications of the sarcoplasmic reticulum and corresponds to the rapidly-exchangeable fraction.

The inotropic action on cardiac muscle of a wide variety of drugs can be explained with reference to their effect on Ca^{2+} exchange within this system. Thus the negative inotropic effect of sodium pentobarbitone on heart muscle is well recognised. As is shown by the record reproduced in Fig. 9, a dose of pentobarbitone (100 μM) which halved the tension developed by dog papillary muscle during regular contraction, abolished the 'staircase effect', so that an increase in the frequency with which contraction was initiated no longer resulted in a positive inotropic response.

Results shown in Fig. 10 may provide an explanation for this finding, because they show that this same dose of sodium pentobarbitone abolished the increase in $^{45}Ca^{2+}$ influx which normally accompanies a reduction in the interval separating successive beats. Hence the effect of sodium pentobarbitone on Ca^{45} influx paralleled its effect on the 'staircase' phenomenon.

Other data included in Fig. 9 indicate, however, that post-stimulation potentiation persisted in the presence of this dose of sodium pentobarbitone, even though the 'staircase' effect is abolished. Sodium pentobarbitone reduces the rate at which Ca^{2+} is accumulated by isolated microsomal fractions[34] so that the pause between successive beats, which would necessarily result

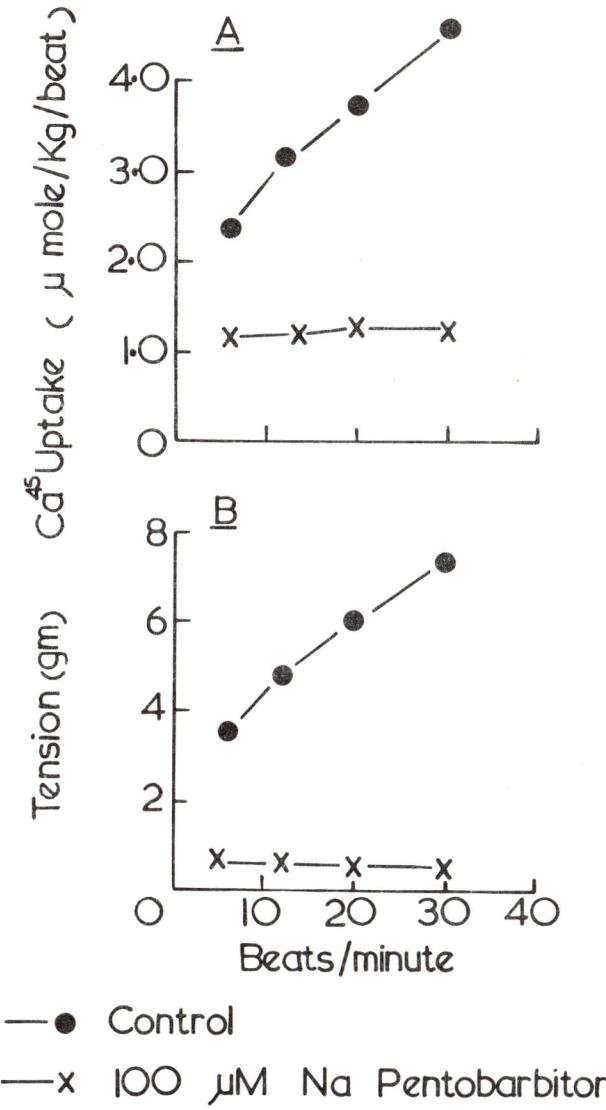

Fig. 10. Effect of 100 μM sodium pentobarbitone on relationship between tension developed during contraction, the frequency with which contraction occurred, and the 'extra' Ca^{2+} influx associated with an altered frequency of contraction. Experiments were performed with dog trabecular muscle immersed in Tyrode's solution at 35° C.

in additional time being available for Ca^{2+} to be accumulated for release, could still result in more Ca^{2+} being available for release during subsequent excitations than would have occurred if the interval separating successive beats had not been prolonged.

If sodium pentobarbitone is taken as an example of a drug which affects the Ca^{2+} influx associated with membrane depolarization, as well as Ca^{2+} exchange (uptake and binding) by the sarcoplasmic reticulum, then ischaemia with its accompanying hypoxia provides an example of a condition which results in a marked reduction in the tension developed during contraction and which cannot be accounted for simply in terms of an altered rate of Ca^{2+} uptake by the sarcoplasmic reticulum.[54] The use of La^{3+} to displace Ca^{2+} bound to extracellular, membrane-located, anionic binding sites[92] has shown that the amount of Ca^{2+} bound to extracellular, membrane-located sites is reduced as the result of hypoxia (Fig. 11). This effect of hypoxia on the Ca^{2+} binding capacity of extracellular superficially-located sites may be associated with the marked reduction in tension developed after relatively **short** periods of hypoxia. After **prolonged** periods of hypoxia the Ca^{2+} accumulating activity of the sarcoplasmic reticulum (isolated as the microsomal fraction) is impaired.

Many drugs which have either positive or negative inotropic effects on heart muscle have been shown to influence Ca^{2+} exchange in heart muscle. These include ouabain,[20, 21, 39, 42, 82] glucagon,[14, 55] catecholamines[14, 22] and others (see ref. 52 for bibliography). In addition to the effect that adrenaline has on Ca^{2+} exchangeability within the sarcoplasmic reticulum[16, 87] it

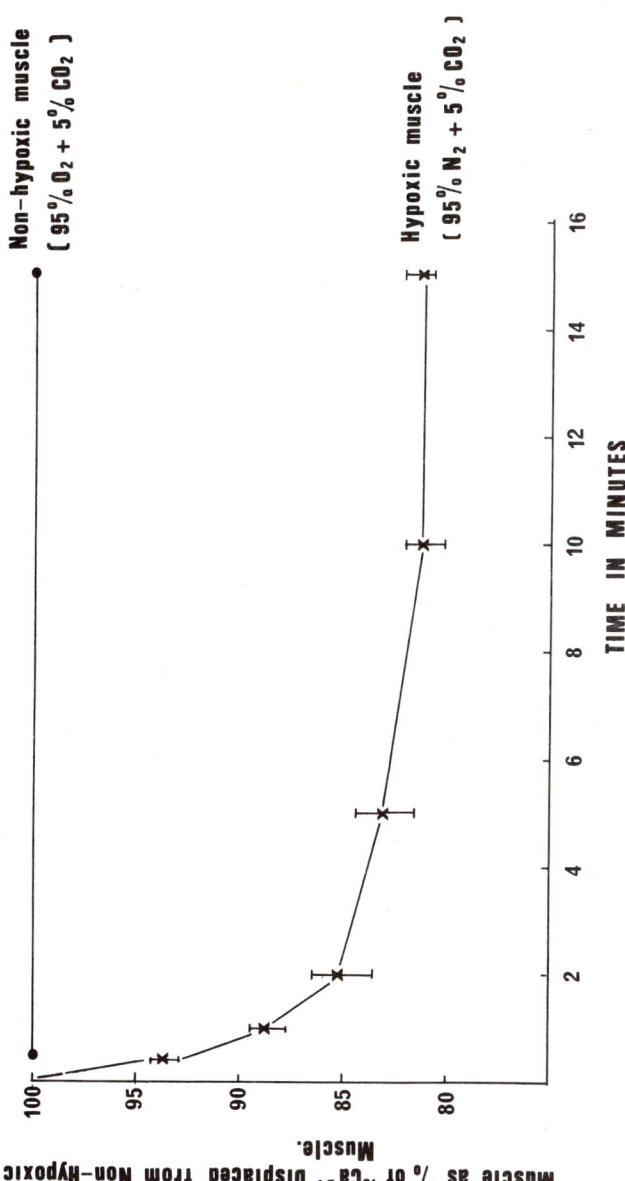

Fig. 11. Effect of 10 minutes anoxia (95% N_2 + 5% CO_2) on the Ca^{2+} displaced by La^{3+} from dog trabecular muscle. La^{3+} was used to displace Ca^{2+} bound to extracellular membrane-located anionic binding sites.

apparently enhances the Ca^{2+} influx associated with the action potential.

Carmeliet and Vereecke[8] were able to show that Mn^{2+} and the β-adrenergic blocking drugs blocked this effect of adrenaline on Ca^{2+} influx. Possibly many of the drugs which effect a change in Ca^{2+} uptake and exchange do so via cyclic 3'5'-AMP. Cyclic 3'5'-AMP is present in sarcoplasmic reticulum fractions isolated from heart muscle[15] and recent investigations[87] have shown cyclic 3' 5'-AMP to have a **direct** effect on Ca^{2+} exchange.

VI. CONCLUSION

In conclusion, the cellular exchange of Ca^{2+} in heart muscle is complex. The development of tension in response to excitation involves an inward-displacement of Ca^{2+} from the extra- to the intracellular phase, and the displacement of Ca^{2+} from superficially-located sites. The sarcoplasmic reticulum, together with its specialized extensions, may provide the sites at which Ca^{2+} can be accumulated and stored for release during subsequent excitation. The close proximity of the transverse tubules and the longitudinal reticulum provides some basis for the hypothesis that the effect of membrane depolarization may be directly translated to the longitudinal reticulum, to effect a release of Ca^{2+}. Changes in the concentration of Ca^{2+} accumulated at the superficially-located sites parallel the changes in developed tension. The amount of Ca^{2+} stored at these intracellular but superficially-located sites depends upon a balance between the extracellular $Ca^{2+}/(Na^+)^2$, the charge transfer carried by Ca^{2+} during preceding depolarizations and the rate of Ca^{2+} efflux. The action of many inotropically-active drugs can be accounted for in terms of their effect on the exchange of Ca^{2+} within this system.

References

1. Antoni, H., Jacob, R. and Kaufmann, R. (1969). Mechanische Reaktionen des Frosch- und Saugetiermyokards bei Veranderung der Aktionspontential-Dauer durch konstante Gleichstromimpulse. Pflüg. Arch. ges. Physiol., **306**, 33.

2. Beeler, G.W., Jr. and Reuter, H. (1970a). Membrane calcium current in ventricular myocardial fibres. J. Physiol., **207**, 191.

3. Beeler, G.W., Jr. and Reuter, H. (1970b). The relation between membrane potential, membrane currents, and activation of contraction in ventricular myocardial fibres. J. Physiol., **207**, 211.

4. Bennett, H.S. and Porter, K. (1953). An electron microscope study of sectioned breast muscle of the domestic fowl. Amer. J. Anat., **93**, 61.

5. Bianchi, C.P. (1961). The effect of caffeine on radiocalcium movement in frog sartorius. J. gen. Physiol., **44**, 845.

6. Blaustein, M.P. and Hodgkin, A.L. (1969). The effect of cyanide on the efflux of calcium from squid axons. J. Physiol., **200**, 497.

7. Carlson, F.D. (1963). The mechanochemistry of muscular contraction: A critical revaluation of in-vitro studies. Prog. biophys. molec. Biol., **13**, 262.

8. Carmeliet, E. and Vereecke, J. (1969). Adrenaline and the plateau phase of the cardiac action potential. Pflüg. Arch. ges. Physiol., **313**, 300.

9. Constantin, L.L., Franzini-Armstrong, C. and Podolsky, R.J. (1965). Localization of calcium-accumulating structures in atrial muscle fibres. Science, **147**, 158.

10   Coraboeuf, E. (1968). Effects of some inhibitors of ionic permeabilities on ventricular action potential and contraction of rat and guinea pig hearts. J. Electrocard., **1**, 19.

11   Davies, R.E. (1964). Adenosine triphosphate breakdown during single muscle contraction. Proc. Roy. Soc., Series B, **160**, 480.

12   Ditmer, D.S. and Grebe, R.M. (Eds.) (1959). Chemical composition of the heart. In 'Handbook of Circulation', p. 1, Saunders, Philadelphia.

13   Ebashi, S. and Endo, M. (1968). Calcium ion and muscle contraction. Prog. biophys. molec. Biol., **18**, 123.

14   Entman, M.L., Levy, G.S. and Epstein, S.E. (1969). Mechanism of action of epinephrine and glucagon on the canine heart: Evidence for increase in sarcotubular calcium stores mediated by cyclic 3'5' AMP. Circ. Res., **25**, 429.

15   Entman, M.L., Levy, G.S. and Epstein, S.E. (1969). Demonstration of adenyl cyclase in canine cardiac sarcoplasmic reticulum. Biochem. Biophys. Res. Com., **35**, 728.

16   Fahrenbach, W.H. (1965). Sarcoplasmic reticulum: Ultrastructure of the triadic function. Science, **147**, 1308.

17   Fawcett, D.W. and McNutt, N.S. (1969). The ultrastructure of the cat myocardium. I. Ventricular papillary muscle. J. Cell Biol., **42**, 1.

18   Forssmann, W.G. and Girardier, L. (1970). A study of the T system in rat heart. J. Cell Biol., **44**, 1.

19   Fuchs, F. and Briggs, F.N. (1968) The site of calcium binding in relation to the activation of myofibrillar contraction. J. gen. Physiol., **51**, 655.

20   Gertz, E.W., Hess, M.L., Lain, R.F. and Briggs, F.N. (1967) Activity of the vesicular calcium pump in the spontaneously failing heart-lung preparation. Circ. Res., **20**, 477.

21   Govier, W.C. and Holland, W.C. (1965). The relationship between atrial contractions and the effect of ouabain on contractile strength and calcium exchange in rabbit atria. J. Pharmacol., **148**, 284.

22   Grossman, A. and Furchgott, R.F. (1964). The effect of various drugs on calcium exchange in the isolated guinea-pig left auricle. J. Pharmacol., **145**, 162.

23   Grossman, A. and Furchgott, R.F. (1964). The effects of frequency of stimulation and calcium concentration on Ca^{45} exchange and contractility in the isolated guinea pig auricle. J. Pharmacol., **143**, 120.

24   Hartshorne, D.J. and Mueller, H. (1967). Separation and recombination of the ethylene glycol bis-(B-aminoethyl ether)-N, N-tetraacetic acid-sensitizing factor obtained from a low ionic strength extract of natural actomyosin. J. biol. Chem., **242**, 3089.

25   Hasselbach, W. (1964). Relaxation and the sarcotubular calcium pump. Fed. Proc., **23**, 909.

26   Hoffman, B.F. and Cranefield, P.F. (1960). 'Electrophysiology of the Heart'. pp. 1-20. McGraw Hill, New York.

27   Huxley, A.F. (1959). Local activation in muscle. Ann. N.Y. Acad. Sci., **81**, 446.

28   Huxley, H.E. (1969). The mechanism of muscular contraction. Science, **164**, 1356.

29   Huxley, A.F. and Taylor, R.E. (1958). Local activation of striated muscle fibres. J. Physiol., **144**, 425.

30   Katz, A.M. (1970). Contractile proteins of the heart. Physiol. Rev., **50**, 63.

31   Katz, A.M. and Repke, D.I. (1967). Quantitative aspects of dog cardiac microsomal calcium binding and calcium uptake. Circ. Res., **21**, 153.

32   Kavaler, F. (1959). Membrane depolarization as a cause of tension development in mammalian ventricular muscle. Amer. J. Physiol., **197**, 968.

33 Koch-Weser, J. and Blinks, J.R. (1963). The influence of the interval between beats on myocardial contractility. Pharmacol. Rev., **15**, 601.

34 Lain, R.F., Hess, M.L., Gertz, E.W. and Briggs, F.N. (1968). Calcium uptake activity of canine myocardial sarcoplasmic reticulum in the presence of anaesthetic agents. Circ. Res., **23**, 597.

35 Langer, G.A. (1964). Kinetic studies of calcium distribution in ventricular muscle of the dog. Circ. Res., **15**, 393.

36 Langer, G.A. (1965). Calcium exchange in dog ventricular muscle: relation to frequency of contraction and maintenance of contractility. Circ. Res., **17**, 79.

37 Langer, G.A. (1968). Ion fluxes in cardiac excitation and contraction and their relation to myocardial contractility. Physiol. Rev., **48**, 708.

38 Langer, G.A. and Brady, A.J. (1963). Calcium flux in the mammalian ventricular myocardium. J. gen. Physiol., **46**, 703.

39 Langer, G.A. and Serena, S.D. (1970). Effects of strophanthidin upon contraction and ionic exchange in rabbit ventricular myocardium: relation to control active state. J. mol. cell. Cardiol., **1**, 65.

40 Lee, K.S., Ladinsky, H., Choi, S.J. and Kasuya, Y. (1966). Studies on the in vitro interaction of electrical stimulation and Ca^{2+} movement in sarcoplasmic reticulum. J. gen. Physiol., **49**, 689.

41 Locke, F.S. and Rosenheim, O. (1907). Contributions to the physiology of the isolated heart. The consumption of dextrose by mammalian cardiac muscle. J. Physiol., **36**, 213.

42 Lullmann, H. and Holland, W. (1962). Influence of ouabain on an exchangeable calcium fraction, contractile force, and resting tension of guinea pig atria. J. Pharmacol., **137**, 186.

43 Luttgau, H.C. and Niedergerke, R. (1958). The antagonism between Ca and Na ions in the frog's heart. J. Physiol., **143**, 486.

44 Martonosi, A. and Feretos, R. (1964). Sarcoplasmic reticulum. 1. The uptake of Ca^{2+} by sarcoplasmic reticulum fragments. J. biol. Chem., **239**, 648.

45 Mascher, D. and Peper, K. (1969). Two components of inward current in myocardial muscle fibres. Pflüg. Arch. ges. Physiol., **307**, 190.

46 Mines, G.R. (1913). On functional analysis by the action of electrolytes. J. Physiol., **46**, 188.

47 Morad, M. and Trautwein, W. (1968). The effect of the duration of the action potential on contraction in the mammalian heart muscle. Pflüg. Arch. ges. Physiol., **299**, 66.

48 Muller, P. (1966). Lokale Konstraktionsauslosung am Herzmuskel. Helv. physiol. acta, **24**, C106-112C.

49 Nayler, W.G. (1963). Effect of caffeine on cardiac contractile activity and radiocalcium movement. Amer. J. Physiol., **204**, 969.

50 Nayler, W.G. (1966). Influx and efflux of calcium in the physiology of muscle contraction. J. clin. Orthop. rel. Res., **46**, 157.

51 Nayler, W.G. (1967). Calcium exchange in cardiac muscle: a basic mechanism of drug action. Amer. Heart J., **73**, 379.

52 Nayler, W.G. (1967). Some factors involved in the maintenance and regulation of cardiac contractility. Circ. Res., Supp. III, **21**, 213.

53 Nayler, W.G. and Merrillees, N.C.R. (1964). Some observations on the fine structure and metabolic activity of normal and glycerinated ventricular muscle of toad. J. Cell Biol., **22**, 533.

54 Nayler, W.G., Stone, J., Carson, V. and Chipperfield, D. (1970). Effect of ischaemia on cardiac contractility and calcium exchangeability. J. cell. molec. Cardiol. (submitted).

55 Nayler, W.G., McInnes, I., Chipperfield, D., Carson, V. and Daile, P. (1970). The effect of glucagon on calcium exchangeability, coronary blood flow, myocardial function and high energy phosphate stores. J. Pharmacol., **171**, 265.

56   Nelson, D.A. and Benson, E.S. (1963). On the structural continuities of the transverse tubular system of rabbit and human myocardial cells. J. Cell Biol., **16**, 297.

57   Niedergerke, R. (1956). The 'staircase' phenomenon and the action of calcium on the heart. J. Physiol., **134**, 569.

58   Niedergerke, R. (1956). The potassium chloride contracture of the heart and its modification by calcium. J. Physiol., **134**, 584.

59   Niedergerke, R. (1957). The rate of action of calcium ions on the contraction of the heart. J. Physiol., **138**, 506.

60   Niedergerke, R. (1959). Calcium and the activation of contraction. Experientia, **15**, 128.

61   Niedergerke, R. (1963). Movement of Ca in beating ventricles of the frog heart. J. Physiol., **167**, 551.

62   Niedergerke, R. and Harris, E.J. (1957). Accumulation of calcium (or strontium) under conditions of increasing contractility. Nature, Lond., **179**, 1068.

63   Niedergerke, R. and Orkand, R.K. (1966). The dual effect of calcium on the action potential of the frog's heart. J. Physiol., **184**, 291.

64   Orkand, R.F. (1968). Facilitation of heart muscle contraction and its dependence on external calcium and sodium. J. Physiol., **196**, 311.

65   Page, E. (1968). Correlations between electron microscopic and physiological observations on heart muscle. J. gen. Physiol., **51**, 211S-220S.

66   Palmer, R.F. and Posey, V.A. (1957). Ion effects on calcium accumulation by cardiac sarcoplasmic reticulum. J. gen. Physiol., **50**, 2085.

67   Peachey, L.D. (1965). The sarcoplasmic reticulum and transverse tubules of the frog's sartorius. J. Cell Biol., **25**, 209.

68 Pease, D.C., Jenden, D.J. and Howell, J.N. (1965). Calcium uptake in glycerol-extracted rabbit psoas muscle fibres. II. Electron microscopic localization at uptake sites. J. cell. comp. Physiol., **65**, 141.

69 Podolsky, R.J. (1965). The role of calcium in the contractile cycle of muscle. In 'First Symposium on Muscle Structure and Function'. pp. 125-130. Paul, W.M. et al. (Eds.). Pergamon Press, London.

70 Pool, P.E. and Sonnenblick, E.H. (1967). The mechanochemistry of cardiac muscle. The isometric contraction. J. gen. Physiol., **50**, 951.

71 Porter, K.R. (1961). The sarcoplasmic reticulum. Its recent history and present status. J.biophys.biochem.Cytol., **10**, Supp. 4, 219.

72 Portzehl, H., Caldwell, P.C. and Ruegg, J.C. (1964). The dependence of contraction and relaxation of muscle fibres from the crab 'Maia squinado' on the internal concentration of free calcium ions. Biochim. biophys. acta, **79**, 581.

73 Rayns, D.G., Simpson, F.O. and Bertaud, W.S. (1968). Surface features of straited muscle. I. Guinea-pig cardiac muscle. J. Cell Sci., **3**, 467.

74 Reuter, H. (1967). The dependence of slow inward current in Purkinje fibres on the extracellular calcium concentration. J. Physiol., **192**, 479.

75 Reuter, H. (1968). Slow inactivation of currents in cardiac Purkinje fibres. J. Physiol., **197**, 233.

76 Reuter, H. and Scholz, H. (1968). Uber den Einfluss der extracellularen Ca-Konzentration auf Membranpotential und Kontraktion isolierter Herzpraparate bei gradurierter Depolarisation. Pflüg. Arch. ges. Physiol., **300**, 87.

77 Reuter, H. and Sietz, H. (1968). The dependence of calcium efflux from cardiac muscle on temperature and external ion composition. J. Physiol., **195**, 451.

78 Revel, J.P. and Karnovsky, M.J. (1967). Hexagonal array of subunits in intercellular junctions of the mouse heart and liver. J.Cell Biol., **33**, C7-C12.

79 Ringer, S. (1883). A further contribution regarding the influence of direct constituents of the blood on the contractions of the heart. J.Physiol., **4**, 29.

80 Rosin, H. and Farah, A. (1955). Post-stimulation of contractility in the isolated auricle of the rabbit. Amer.J. Physiol., **180**, 75.

81 Rostgaard, J. and Behnke, O. (1965). Fine structural localization of adenine nucleoside phosphatase activity in the sarcoplasmic reticulum and the T system of rat myocardium. J.Ultrastruct.Res., **12**, 579.

82 Sabatini-Smith, S. and Holland, W.C. (1967). Effects of temperature and ouabain on the rate of action of calcium on atrial tissue. J.Pharmacol., **158**, 22.

83 Sandow, A. (1952). Excitation-contraction coupling in muscular response. Yale J.Biol.Med., **25**, 176.

84 Sandow, A. (1965). Excitation-contraction coupling in skeletal muscle. Pharmacol.Rev., **17**, 265.

85 Scales, B. and McIntosh, D.A.D. (1968). Studies on the radiocalcium uptake and adenosine triphosphatases of skeletal and cardiac sarcoplasmic reticulum fragments. J.Pharmacol., **160**, 249.

86 Shelburne, J.C., Serena, S.D. and Langer, G.A. (1967). The rate-tension staircase in rabbit ventricular muscle: relation to ionic exchange. Amer.J.Physiol., **213**, 1115.

87 Shinebourne, E. and White, R. (1970). Cyclic AMP and calcium uptake of sarcoplasmic reticulum in relation to increased rate of relaxation under the influence of catecholamines. Cardiovasc.Res., **4**, 194.

88 Simpson, F.O. (1965). The transverse tubular system in mammalian myocardial cells. Amer.J.Anat., **117**, 1.

89 Simpson, F.O. and Oertelis, S.J. (1962). The fine structure of sheep myocardial cells, sarcolemmal invaginations and the transverse tubular systems. J. Cell Biol., **12**, 91.

90 Simpson, F.O. and Rayns, D.G. (1968). The relationship between the transverse tubular system and other tubules at the Z disc level of myocardial cells in the ferret. Amer. J. Anat., **122**, 193.

91 Staley, N.A. and Benson, E.S. (1968). The ultrastructure of frog ventricular cardiac muscle and its relationship to mechanisms of excitation-contraction coupling. J. Cell Biol., **38**, 99.

92 Breeman, C. van and McNaughton, C. (1970). The separation of cell membrane calcium transport from extracellular calcium exchange in vascular smooth muscle. Biochem. biophys. Res. Com., **39**, 567.

93 Weber, A. (1959). On the role of calcium in the activity of adenosine 5-triphosphate hydrolysis by actomyosin. J. biol. Chem., **234**, 2764.

94 Weber, A. and Herz, R. (1963). The binding of calcium to actomyosin systems in relation to their biological activity. J. biol. Chem., **238**, 599.

95 Weber, A., Herz, R. and Reiss, I. (1964). The regulation of myofibrillar activity by calcium. Proc. Roy. Soc., Series B, **160**, 489.

96 Wiedmann, S. (1958). Electrical events underlying the cardiac contraction. In 'Circulation', pp. 100-109. McMichael, J. (Ed.). Blackwell, Oxford.

97 Wilbrandt, W. von and Koller, H. (1948). Die Calciumwirkung am Froschherzen als Funktion des Ionengleichgewichts zwischen Zellmembran und Umgebung. Helv. physiol. acta, **6**, 208.

98 Winegrad, S. (1961). The possible role of calcium in excitation-contraction coupling of heart muscle. Circulation, **24**, 523.

99 Winegrad, S. (1970). The intracellular site of calcium activation of contraction in frog skeletal muscle. J. gen. Physiol., **55**, 77.

100 Winegrad, S. and Shanes, A.M. (1962). Calcium flux and contractility in guinea pig atria. J. gen. Physiol., **45**, 371.

101 Wood, E.H., Heppner, R.L. and Wiedmann, S. (1969). Inotropic effects of electric currents. I. Positive and negative effects of constant electric currents or current impulses applied during cardiac action potentials. II. Hypothesis: Calcium movements, excitation-contraction coupling and inotropic effects. Circ. Res., **24**, 209.

CALCIUM AND THE SARCOPLASMIC RETICULUM

ARNOLD SCHWARTZ

Division of Myocardial Biology, Baylor College
of Medicine, Houston, Texas 77025

I. INTRODUCTION AND HISTORY

Since the time of Ringer, it has been well accepted that calcium is required to maintain appropriate contraction in heart muscle. Furthermore, it seems appropriate to regard calcium as a key cation in contraction of all muscles. In the case of vertebrate skeletal muscles, a variety of experiments have resulted in the conclusion that the calcium involved in activation of the contractile system arises from an intracellular source. It is apparent that normal skeletal muscle contraction can be elicited in the absence of external calcium and, moreover, the twitch tension of vertebrate skeletal muscle is not appreciably changed by alterations in extracellular calcium.[8] It is quite apparent, however, that the maintenance of contractile force in heart muscle does require specific changes in external calcium ion concentration.[16,17]

Moreover, external calcium ion maintains twitch tension and is required for the slow and incomplete development of the active state by a single stimulus.[3] Furthermore, it appears that Sr^{++} can substitute for calcium in Ringer's solution used for excised frog heart.[27] It appears that the sensitivity of the contractile system of heart muscle to Sr^{++} is very much the same as that to calcium. This is very much unlike the contractile system of skeletal muscle. All of this and other evidence strongly suggests that calcium is required for the activation of the contractile system of the heart, and that it comes directly from the extracellular medium. Unfortunately, the amount of calcium ion entering the heart muscle fiber, namely about 3×10^{-6} M/single twitch,[20] is too small to account for the total activation of the contractile system, if the calcium requirement of heart is similar to that of skeletal muscle. It appears probable, therefore, that calcium arises both from extracellular sources and from intracellular storage sites.

It is quite clear that skeletal muscles employ an intracellular store of calcium and that this calcium probably arises from specific areas of the sarcoplasmic reticulum, possibly from the terminal cisternae (Fig. 1). The main question at the beginning of 1950 was: 'What is the enzymatic mechanism responsible for intracellular calcium metabolism in muscle such that both contraction and relaxation can occur at appropriate rates, consistent with physiological requirements?' In 1951, B.B. Marsh published a short note in 'Nature'[18] describing the isolation of a 'relaxing factor'. The factor was derived from an aqueous extract of skeletal muscle

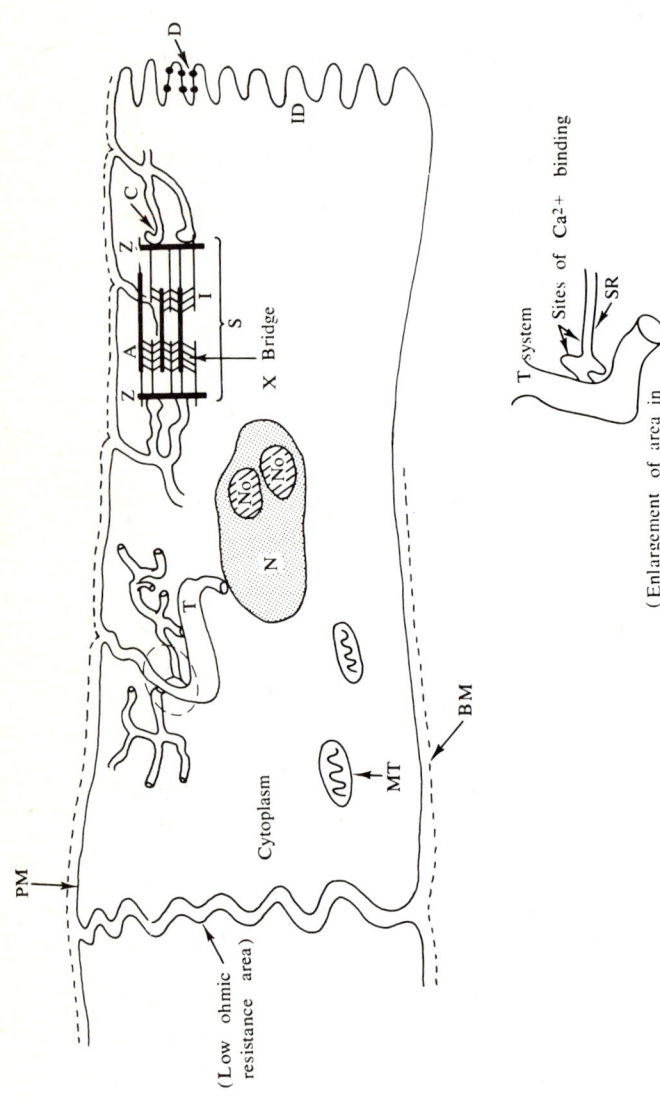

Fig. 1. Diagrammatic sketch of cardiac muscle cell. PM, plasma membrane; BM, basement membrane; T, T-system; C, cisterna of SR; MT, mitochondrion; S, sarcomere of myofibril; I, I band of sarcomere (actin); A, A band of sarcomere (myosin);(note cross bridges between A and I); N, nucleus; No, nucleolus; ID, intercalated disc; D, desmosome; SR, sarcoplasmic reticulum; Z, Z line (borders one sarcomere). (From Bresnick and Schwartz.[4])

tissue; inclusion of this material in an in vitro system containing myofibrils in the presence of ATP prevented syneresis (super-precipitation). Furthermore, the inhibition of syneresis was overcome by small amounts of calcium. The extract also relaxed glycerol extracted fiber bundles that were previously contracted by the addition of ATP and Mg^{++} ions.[1] Bendall, in 1954,[1] compared the activity of a relatively purified myokinase (adenylate kinase) with the aqueous extract and found that the effects were rather similar. Bendall concluded that myokinase might be the so-called relaxing factor. Thus, the Marsh-Bendall factor was thought of as a soluble material that was capable of inducing relaxation of contracted fibers and that relaxation could be prevented by appropriate concentrations of calcium. Accordingly, the factor became known as 'relaxing factor' and its mechanism appeared to involve some type of interaction with calcium and the contractile elements. In subsequent years, numerous investigators have attempted to isolate this soluble factor from a variety of tissues.[6, 13, 24] A long list of possible substances that could induce relaxation was proposed; among these, perhaps the most fascinating was 3', 5'-cyclic AMP, suggested by the studies of Uchida and Mommaerts.[23] Unfortunately, within a short period, it was shown that this substance was not the elusive relaxing factor.[11]

The search for a soluble relaxing factor was terminated by the discovery that the material which effected relaxation was of particulate origin. This was first disclosed in the work of Ebashi.[7] Fig. 2, taken from Ebashi's work, shows that over 80% of the calcium ion in solution could be bound, in the presence of ATP, by

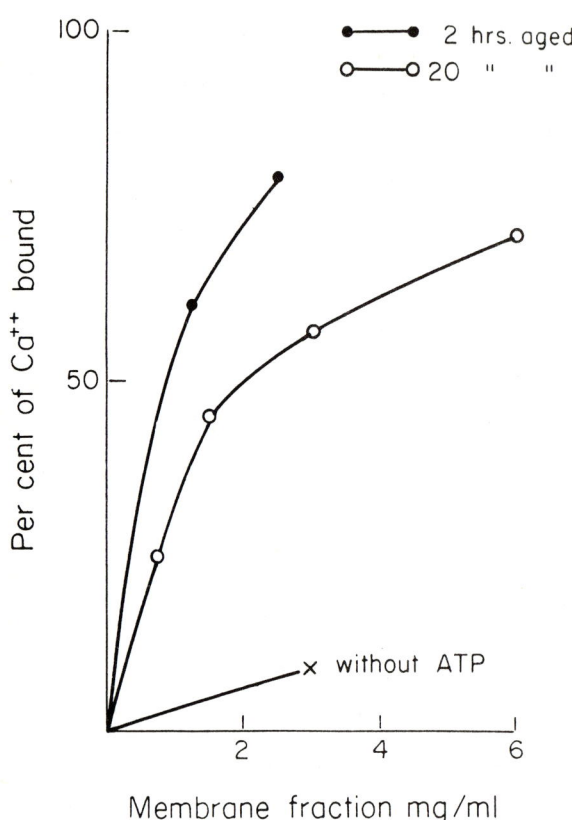

Fig. 2. ATP-dependent calcium ion binding with various concentrations of normal and aged membrane fraction.
(From Ebashi and Lipmann.[7])

a sarcoplasmic reticulum fraction from rabbit skeletal muscle. This was equivalent to approximately 1400-fold concentration of calcium ion in the granules as compared with the surrounding fluid. The discovery was corroborated by Weber and her colleagues,[24] and by all the other investigators active in this field. The particulate relaxing system or factor could not only actively remove calcium from solution, but also could effect relaxation of contracted fibers, and inhibition of contractile fiber-associated ATPase activity simultaneously with the removal of calcium from the vicinity of the myofibrils. Fig. 3 graphically demonstrates these interesting effects.

It was soon found, however, that two types of ATP-dependent calcium accumulation could be shown, with particulate preparations: (1) a rapid binding and subsequent release; and (2) a rapid and extensive accumulation with no release. The former process occurred in the absence of inorganic phosphate or oxalate and the latter in the presence of either oxalate or phosphate. It was soon apparent that the accumulation of calcium in the presence of either oxalate or phosphate was the result of a movement of calcium ions across the vesicular grana and subsequent probable precipitation of calcium phosphate or calcium oxalate within the vesicles. The accumulation process in the absence of a precipitating ion is referred to as **binding** and accumulation in the presence of a participating anion is referred to as **uptake.** The important studies of Hasselbach and his colleagues established that, during the process of calcium uptake, an increased calcium-dependent ATPase activity known as 'extra splitting' took place. This extra splitting was

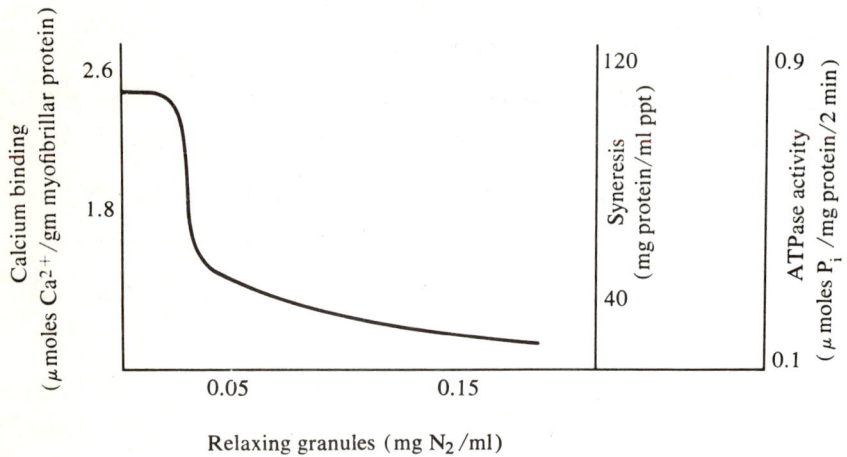

Fig. 3. Effect of SR (relaxing system) on calcium binding, syneresis and ATPase of myofibrils. Incubation time: 130 seconds. Medium: $^{45}CaCl_2$, 0.02 mM, ATP-Mg, 4 mM, oxalate, 1 mM, myofibrils, protein = 1.98 mg/ml.

(From Weber et al.[25, 26] and Bresnick and Schwartz.[4])

completely inhibited by the same concentrations of salyrgan (salicyl-hydroxy mercuri-methoxypropyl-amidoorthoacetate) that inhibited calcium uptake. It is of interest that the so-called basic splitting, which occurs in the absence of oxalate, is insensitive to salyrgan. The parallelism between the storage of calcium in the grana and the activity of the extra ATPase induced Hasselbach to suggest that the extra splitting of ATP represents the source of energy necessary for storage of calcium. This extra splitting appeared to be also accompanied by an ATP-ADP exchange reaction. The basic splitting appeared not to be connected with an ATP-ADP exchange reaction. The relationship between extra splitting, ATP-ADP exchange reaction and calcium uptake is represented in Fig. 4.

As a result of his investigations, Hasselbach suggested that calcium accumulation occurred in a complex manner by means of a carrier present on the outer surface of the granules. Phosphorylation by ATP of the carrier, which occurs presumably on the outer portion of the membrane, greatly increases affinity of the grana for calcium. The calcium complex of the phosphorylated carrier would then diffuse to the inner surface of the granule. There the phosphate group would be split off from the carrier, thereby diminishing the calcium affinity of the carrier. At this time, the bound calcium would be liberated in spite of the comparatively high concentration of calcium inside the grana.[10]

Ebashi has pointed out that studies of calcium accumulation in the presence of oxalate yields very little information concerning mechanism and has suggested that the binding process in the absence

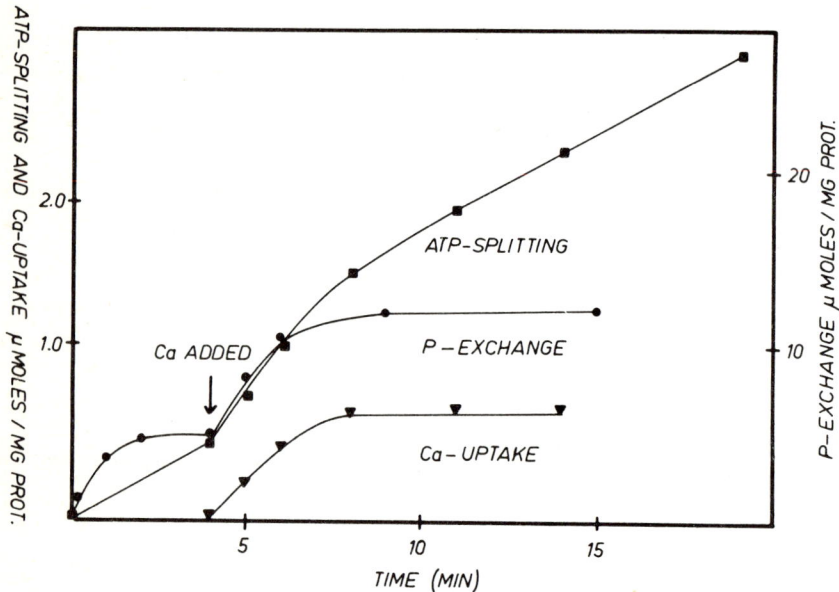

Fig. 4. ATP 'extra' splitting, calcium uptake and phosphate exchange. Mg^{++} = oxalate = ATP = 5.10^{-3} M, μ = 0.1, histidine = 0.01 M, pH = 7.0, T = 20° C, 0.46 mg prot/ml. (From Hasselbach and Makinose.[10])

of oxalate is of primary significance.[6] Thus, at present there are two proposed mechanisms for intracellular calcium accumulation or the sarcoplasmic reticulum, both in skeletal and heart muscle: (1) the active transport of hypothesis of Hasselbach (described above), which is based on the stoichiometry of ATP splitting and calcium uptake; and (2) the two-stage binding and active transport process suggested by Ebashi and his co-workers. The latter suggests that the first step in calcium accumulation involves an ATP-induced conformational change of the membrane before any splitting of ATP occurs. The membrane perturbation results in calcium binding and presumably movement of calcium into the vesicle would then involve ATP hydrolysis, but with unknown stoichiometry. In point of fact, most investigators find difficulty in obtaining definitive stoichiometry between ATP hydrolysis and calcium accumulation.

While a relaxing system in heart similar to that found in skeletal muscle has been isolated and characterized to some extent,[12, 15, 24] the lability and apparent paucity of particulate sarcoplasmic reticulum in most mammalian hearts have prompted investigators to question the complete participation of the sarcoplasmic reticulum relaxing factor in cardiac muscle relaxation. The efforts in our laboratory have been directed towards the isolation of a highly active fraction and the use of rapid spectrophotometric recording procedures in order to answer the question: 'Can intracellular membranes in cardiac muscle bind and release calcium in amounts and in rates consistent with relaxation and possibly contraction?'

II. MATERIALS AND METHODS

I. Isolation[9]

This procedure is a modification of a water extraction proposed by Inesi and his co-workers,[12] but with the use of a rapid shearing device called a Polytron.

II. Methods of assay

A. Millipore filtration.
B. Dual-beam spectrophotometry using murexide.
   1. Rapid vibrating device.
   2. Stopped-flow spectrophotometry.
C. Single-beam stopped-flow spectrophotometry (Durrum spectrophotometer).

III. RESULTS

Figs. 5 and 6 indicate the device employed for spectrophotometric measurements of calcium binding. Fig. 6 indicates the principle of the murexide procedure. This procedure was introduced by Ohnishi and Ebashi,[21] and has proven to be of immense value in studying apparent initial velocity of binding. Fig. 7 compares the calcium binding process between cardiac muscle, white muscle and red muscle using the murexide procedure. Note that in both white and cardiac muscle there is always a release process after equilibrium calcium binding occurs. The nature of this process is unknown, although it is quite

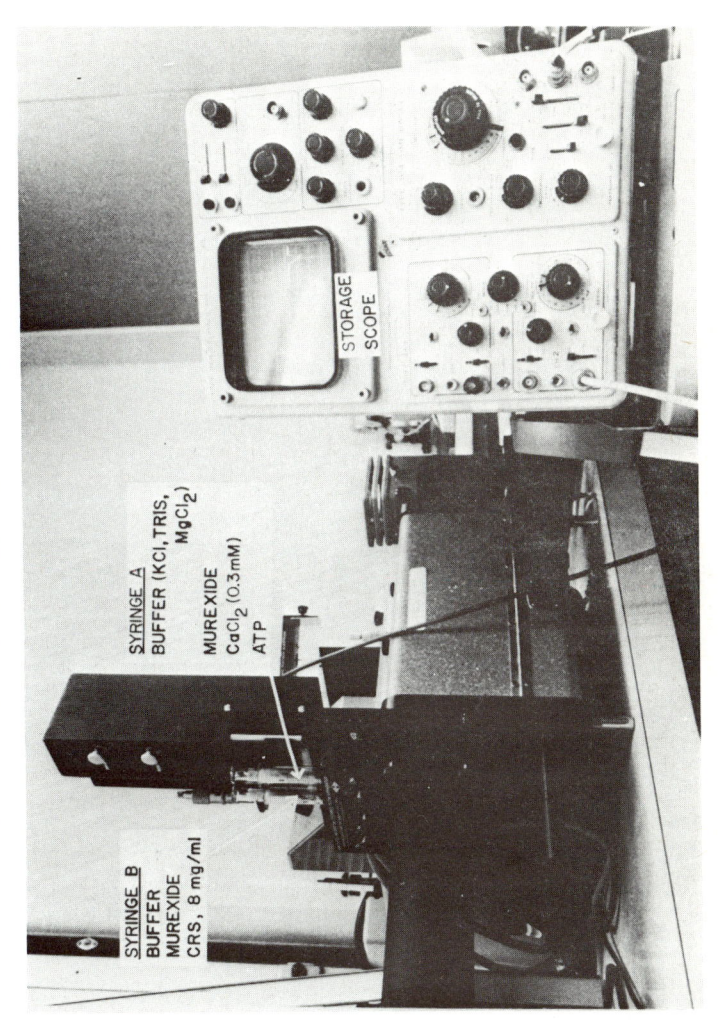

Fig. 5. Device employed for spectrophotometric measurements of calcium binding.

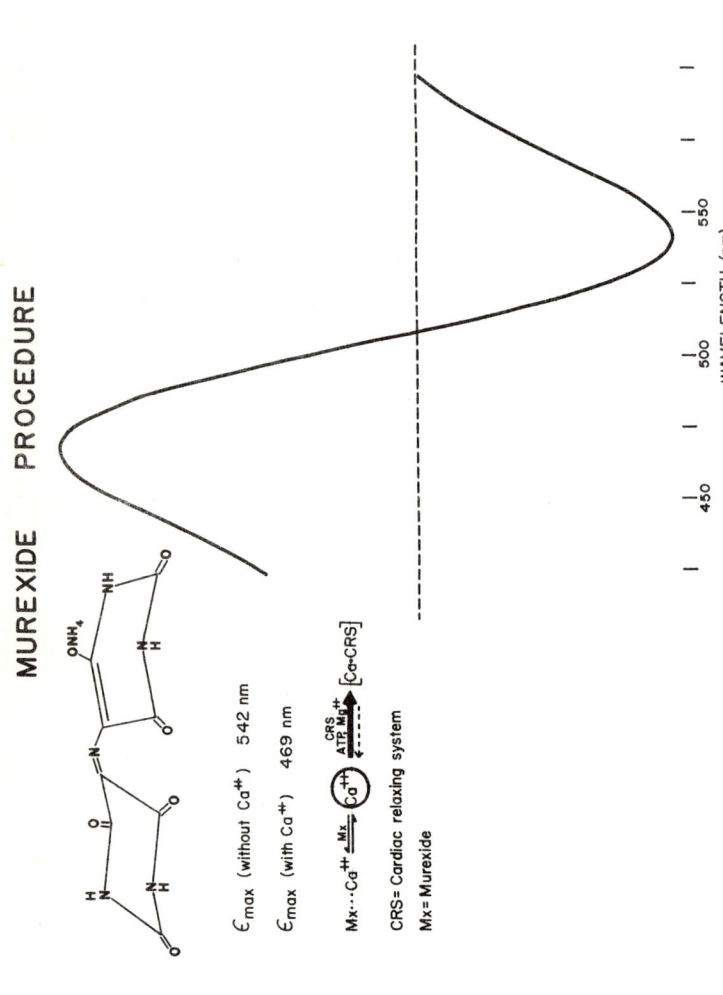

Fig. 6. Principle of murexide procedure to study apparent initial velocity of binding of calcium to cardiac relaxing system. (See Ohnishi and Ebashi.[21])

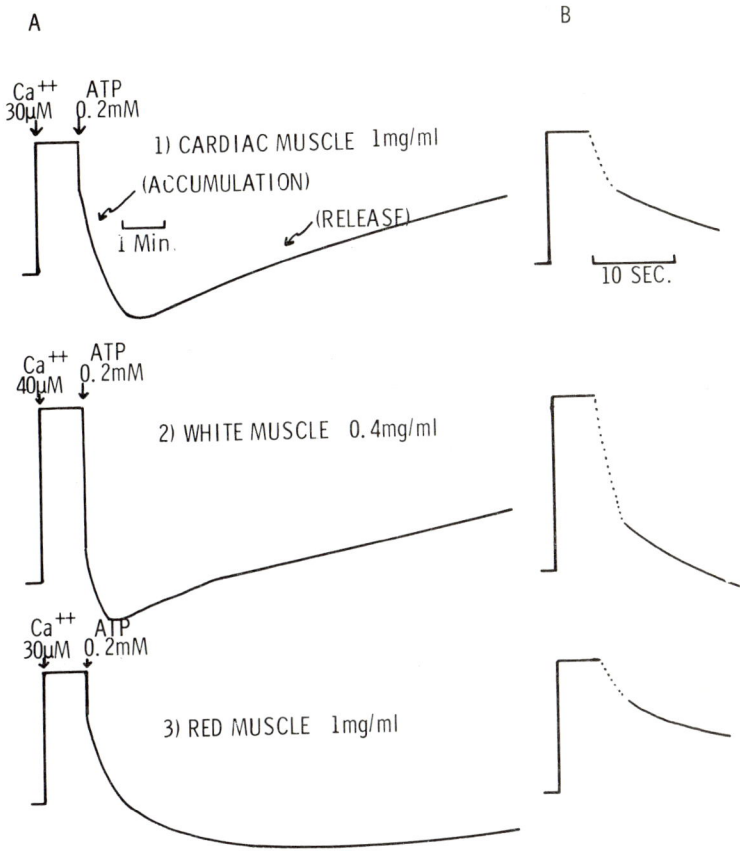

Fig. 7. Rate of Ca^{2+} binding by relaxing preparations from various muscles of rabbit, measured by dual-beam spectrophotometry. Reaction mixture consisted of 100 mM KCl, 10 mM $MgCl_2$, 20 mM Tris-maleate buffer (pH 6.8), 0.3 mM murexide, 0.4-1 mg per ml membrane protein, 30-40 μM Ca^{2+} and 0.2 mM ATP. Incubation at room temperature (about 23° C). A and B are the same, except for different time scales. The ordinate in this figure and in Figs. 3, 4, 6 and 12 represents changes in transmitted light expressed in units of optical density (OD).
(From Harigaya and Schwartz.[9])

characteristic of normal fresh preparations. In the case of red
muscle, the release is seldom noticed. The release process still
occurs in the presence of an ATP regenerating system, which
means that it is more complicated than just limiting amounts of
ATP. Using more rapid methods of recording, namely the introduction of a vibrator into the mixing chamber which permits
measurements in less than three seconds, and stopped-flow
spectrophotometry employing an Aminco-Morrow attachment,
extremely rapid binding rates were obtained using fresh cardiac
relaxing system derived from a variety of mammals (Figs. 8 and
9). Using the Durrum stopped-flow spectrophotometer, which
permits mixing in millisecond ranges, we have been able to
calculate even more rapid apparent initial binding rates (Fig.
10).

The approximate calcium binding constant of the cardiac
relaxing system (the absence of oxalate) is about 5×10^7 M^{-1},
which is higher than the binding constant of calcium for troponin.
This suggests that the in vitro affinity of calcium for CRS is
greater than for troponin. The half-maximal time for calcium
binding in cardiac muscle is probably less than six seconds; the
apparent initial rate of binding in fresh preparations ranges from
130-500 picomoles calcium/mg protein/millisecond. The amount
of binding calculated in 200 milliseconds is 15.5 nanomoles/mg
protein or approximately 50-60 nanomoles calcium/g wet weight
of cardiac muscle assuming a 40% recovery of reticulum. The
procedure employed for isolation of the cardiac relaxing system
was refined to yield a preparation that bound maximally from 60

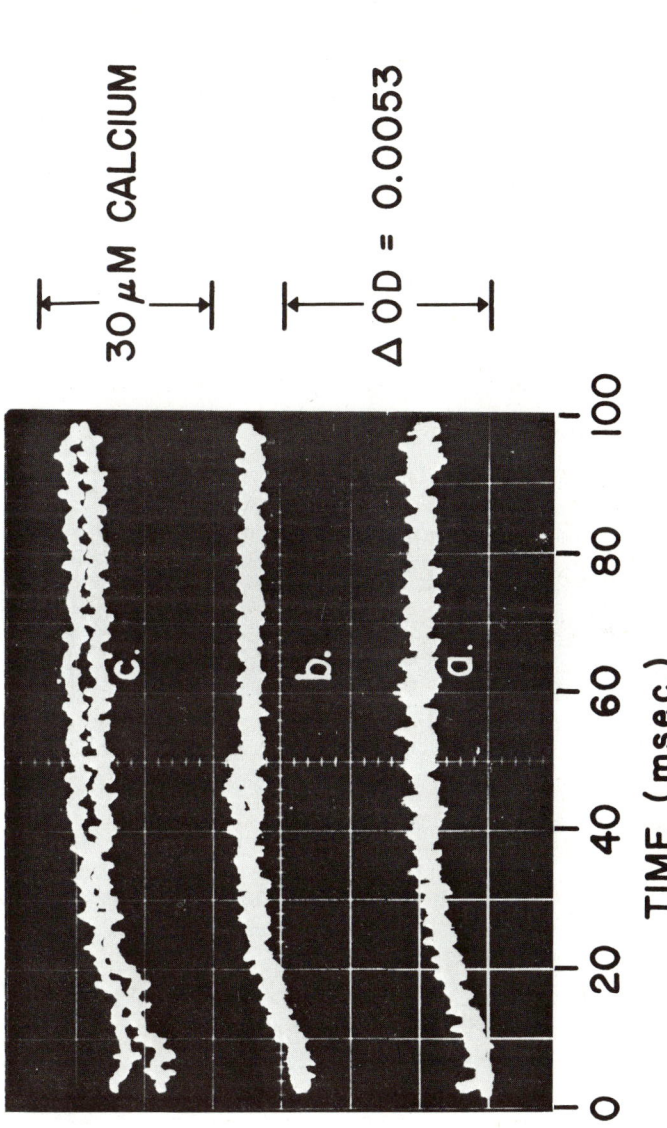

Fig. 8. Calibration of Aminco-Morrow stopped-flow apparatus with Aminco-Chance dual wavelength spectrophotometer. The medium, at 25° C, consisted of 100 mM KCl, 10 mM $MgCl_2$, 20 mM Tris-maleate (pH 6.8), 0.2 mM murexide, 0.8 mg/ml cardiac relaxing system, and (a) no added calcium; (b) 30 μM calcium; and (c) 60 μM calcium. No ATP was present. Oscilloscopic sweep speed was 10 milliseconds/cm. Linearity was achieved after 40 milliseconds. Wavelengths were 507 mμ and 542 mμ. (Amer. J. Physiol., to be published.)

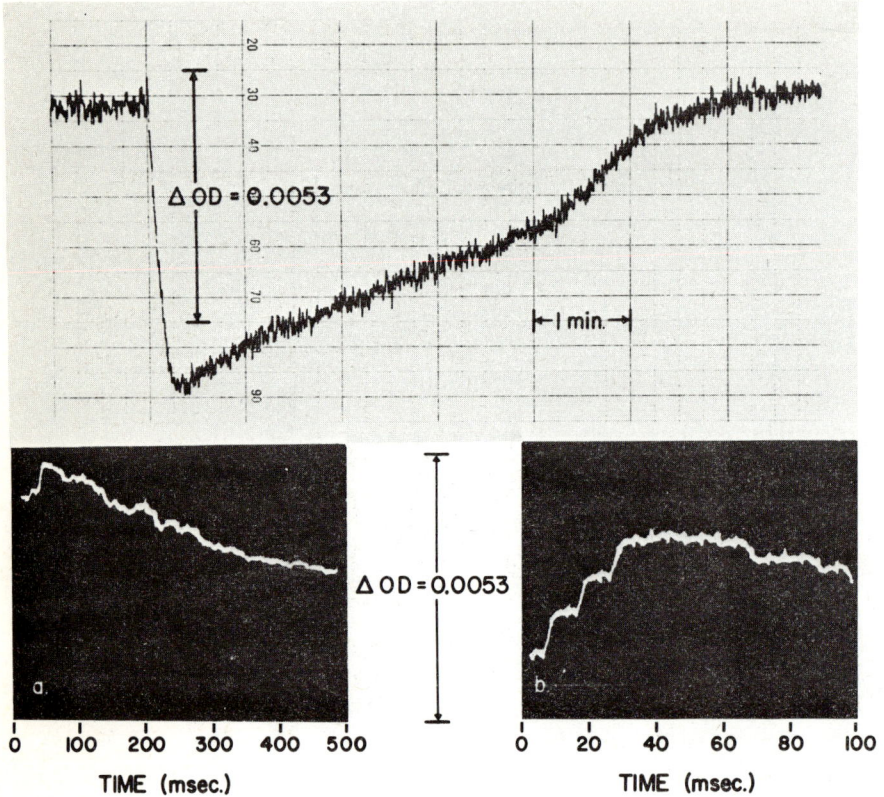

Fig. 9. Calcium binding and release by dog cardiac relaxing system (CRS) measured by Aminco-Chance dual-wavelength spectrophotometer with stopped-flow mixing. The reaction mixture and conditions are the same as in Fig. 8, i.e., 0.8 mg/ml CRS, 30 μM calcium and 0.2 mM ATP. The insets are oscilloscopic traces of initial binding recorded in parallel with the larger paper trace. (A): 50 millisecond/cm sweep speed. (B): 10 millisecond/cm sweep speed. The rising part of the inset traces indicates mixing of reactants. (Amer. J. Physiol., to be published.)

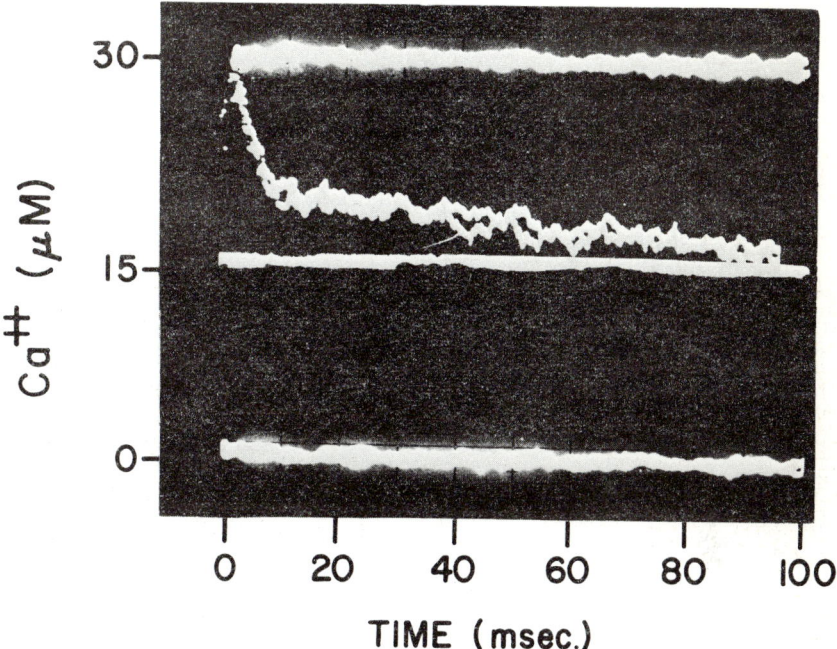

Fig. 10. Calcium binding by canine CRS measured by Durrum Stopped-Flow spectrophotometry. The reaction mixture was as in Fig. 8, i.e., 0.8 mg/ml CRS, 30 μM calcium and 0.2 mM ATP. The linear traces were calibrations in the presence of no added calcium (zero mark), 15 μM calcium, and 30 μM calcium. Each curve represents two consecutive determinations. Oscilloscopic sweep speed was 10 milliseconds/cm. Wavelength was 520 mμ. (Amer. J. Physiol., to be published.)

to 90 nanomoles calcium/mg protein at 25° C. From the well known temperature-dependency of the calcium binding reaction, at body temperature, approximately 100 nanomoles calcium/g of ventricle would be bound in 200 milliseconds (average relaxation time of mammalian ventricle).

The calcium release phenomenon

We have recently found that rapid alteration of proton concentration, employing dual-beam spectrophotometric procedures, produces a reversible and rapid release of calcium. For example, optimal binding pH is around 6.5-6.7. If the pH is changed rapidly from 6.74 to pH 5.94, an increment of binding is noted. If the pH is altered from 6.74 to 7.83, a rapid release of binding occurs. The release of bound calcium at the appropriate pH occurs at a rate which is approximately the same as the binding rate for calcium at the latter's optimal pH (Fig. 11). This phenomenon was noted not only with cardiac muscle relaxing system,

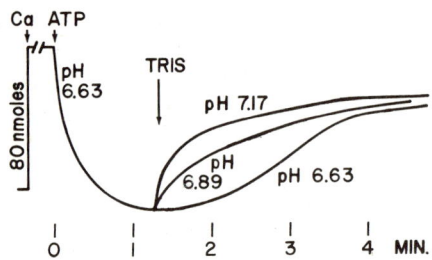

Fig. 11. Effect of rapid pH change on calcium release from isolated cardiac sarcoplasmic reticulum. An Aminco dual-beam spectrophotometer was employed; pH was changed from 6.63 to 6.89 and to 7.17 respectively by injection of either Tris or KOH into the curette. The medium and conditions were similar to those described in Fig. 8. (Amer. J. Physiol., to be published.)

but also with relaxing factor obtained from skeletal muscle and a similar system derived from brain. Perhaps of even greater interest is the following experiment carried out with relaxing system in the presence of native actomyosin:—

> Superprecipitation or syneresis of actomyosin, requiring ATP and calcium, may be conveniently measured by a spectrophotometric procedure developed by Ebashi.[5] In Fig. 12, note that a significant increase of optical density, representing superprecipitation, occurs in the presence of calcium and ATP at pH 7.6, in the absence of sarcoplasmic reticulum. When appropriate amounts of sarcoplasmic reticulum are added at pH 7.6, no noticeable change in syneresis occurs. However, if the same process is carried out at pH 6.2, very little superprecipitation of actomyosin occurs. This is due to the increased affinity of the relaxing system for calcium at lower pH's. When the pH is raised from 6.2 to 7.8 by the addition of KOH or Tris, calcium released from the SR interacts with the actomyosin system and syneresis occurs.

This experiment indicates that proton concentration may be a physiological controller of intracellular calcium availability. It is of interest to speculate that in some pathological conditions, such as ischemic heart disease or congestive heart failure, alterations of intracellular pH cause altered affinity of the sarcoplasmic reticulum. Katz and Hecht[14] recently suggested that the increase of proton concentration usually seen in ischemic heart disease may result in the release of calcium from troponin, which would result in a diminution in the number of actin-myosin interactions.

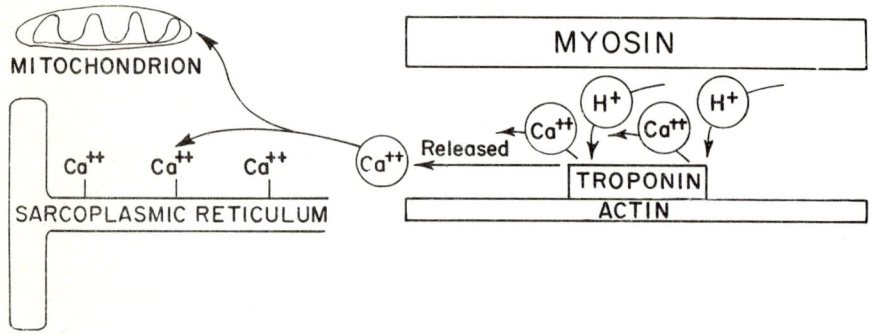

INTRACELLULAR ACIDOSIS DECREASES AFFINITY OF TROPONIN FOR CALCIUM AND INCREASES AFFINITY OF MEMBRANES FOR CALCIUM

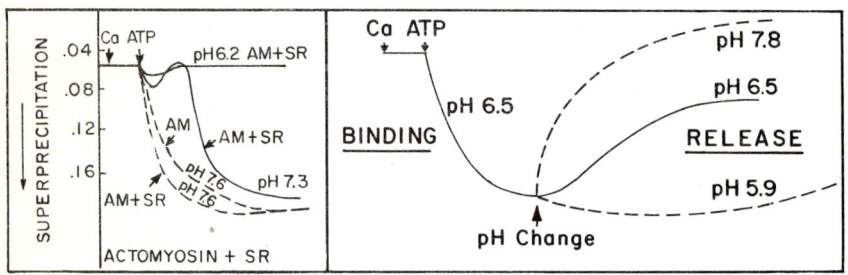

Fig. 12. A diagrammatic representation of one possible molecular mechanism of heart failure. Affinity of sarcoplasmic reticulum (SR) for calcium increases with increasing $[H]^+$ (see right panel). The left panel indicates a combined actomyosin-SR experiment. Isolated native actomyosin was added to a cuvette and optical density increases (which measure superprecipitation) were measured as described. Turbidity change was recorded at 660 nm with continuous mixing by a stationary vibrator. Conditions: 50 mM Tris-maleate-KOH, 4 mM $MgCl_2$, 100 mM KCl, 3 mg actomyosin protein/3 ml and 0.68 mg SR protein/3 ml at 25° C. Line AM = pH 7.6 without SR; line AM + SR = pH 7.6 with SR; line AM + SR = pH 6.5 with SR; line AM + SR = with SR, pH was abruptly changed from 6.2 to 7.3. Note the slight lag and then superprecipitation ensues indicating loss of Ca^{++} from SR to Troponin. (Amer. J. Physiol., to be published.)

We would like to suggest an alternative hypothesis, namely that changes in intracellular pH cause rapid alteration of affinity of intracellular membranes for calcium (Fig. 12).

The cardiac relaxing system in the failing heart

Recently, we have shown that relaxing system isolated from failing human heart exhibits a significantly diminished rate of binding of calcium and almost no release of calcium. These results were duplicated in a cardiomyopathic Syrian hamster model (Figs. 13 and 14).

Digitalis and the cardiac relaxing system

We have found no demonstrable effect, either in vitro or in vivo, of cardiac glycosides on skeletal or cardiac relaxing systems.[2, 22]

IV. DISCUSSION

The described experiments clearly indicate that membrane vesicles, presumably sarcoplasmic reticulum derived from heart, possess the in vitro rate and capacity for binding calcium consistent with a role in muscle relaxation. Estimates of the amounts of calcium required for binding to effect relaxation in vivo range from 60 to 160 nanomoles/g wet weight of tissue,[9, 13] and our preparations fulfill this in vitro.

Preliminary experiments in our laboratory strongly suggest a role for the sarcoplasmic reticulum in the relaxing system in cardiac muscle disease.

"NORMAL" (PRESERVATION CHAMBER)   FAILING (RECIPIENT HEART)

MUREXIDE PROCEDURE

30 μM Ca^{++} 0.2 mM ATP   1 Min   30 μM Ca^{++} 0.2 mM ATP

ΔOD=0.0044   ΔOD=0.0044

rate $_{(5'')}$ = 115.2 n moles Ca / mg protein / min   rate $_{(5'')}$ = 42 n moles Ca / mg protein / min
max binding = 40.3 n moles Ca / mg protein   max binding = 35.2 n moles Ca / mg protein
$t_{1/2}$ = 23 sec $t_{1/2}$ = 70 sec

Spectrophotometric recordings of calcium binding and release by relaxing system from human heart

The downward deflection with ATP addition is the uptake phase. Failing preparations exhibit little or no release phase.

POSSIBLE BIOCHEMICAL CAUSE OF HEART FAILURE

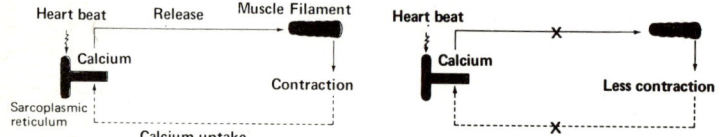

The possible biochemical "lesion" involving the inability of failing "cardiac relaxing system" to sequester and release calcium for the proper contraction and relaxation of the myofibrils

Fig. 13

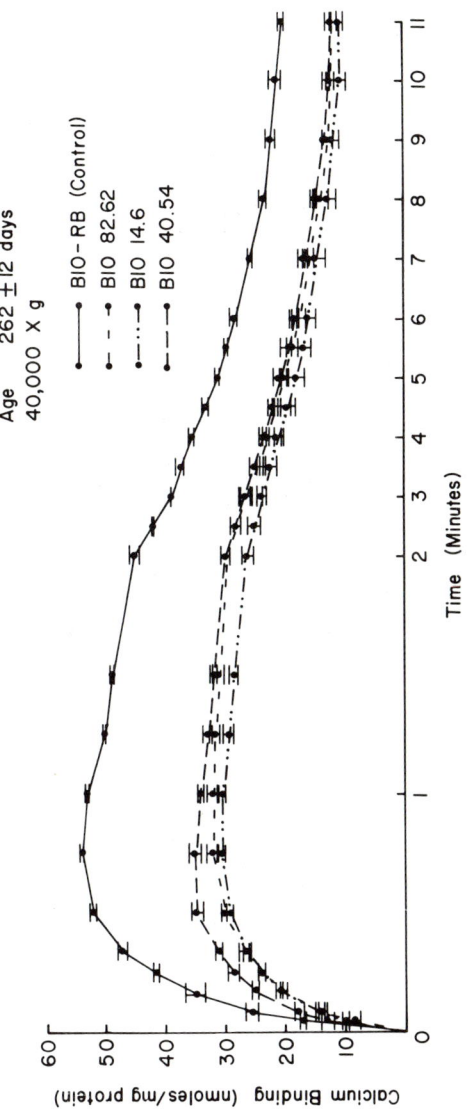

Fig. 14. Calcium binding by 40,000 g (cardiac relaxing system) of myopathic Syrian hamsters of various strains (B10-RB = control; B10 82.62, 14.6, and 40.54 = diseased). All were about 262 days old. Note defective calcium binding by cardiac relaxing system of myopathic strains.

References

1. Bendall, J.R. (1954). The relaxing effect of myokinase on muscle fibers; its identity with the 'Marsh' factor. Proc. Roy. Soc., **142B**, 409.

2. Besch, H.R., jr., Allen, J.C., Glick, G. and Schwartz, A. (1970). Correlation between the inotropic action of ouabain and its effects on subcellular enzyme systems from canine myocardium. J. Pharmacol., **171**, 1.

3. Brady, A.J. (1966). Onset of contractility on cardiac muscle. J. Physiol., **184**, 560.

4. Bresnick, E. and Schwartz, A. (1968). 'Functional Dynamics of the Cell'. Academic Press, New York.

5. Ebashi, S. (1961). Calcium binding activity of vesicular relaxing factor. J. Biochem., **50**, 236.

6. Ebashi, S. and Endo, M. (1968). Calcium ion and muscle contraction. In 'Progress in Biophysics and Molecular Biology'. Butler, J.A.V. and Noble, D. (Eds.), pp. 123-183. Pergamon Press, New York.

7. Ebashi, S. and Lipmann, F. (1962). Adenosine triphosphate linked concentration of calcium ions in a particulate fraction of rabbit muscle. J. Cell Biol., **14**, 389.

8. Frank, G.B. (1962). Utilization of bound calcium in the action of caffeine and certain monovalent cations on skeletal muscle. J. Physiol., **163**, 254.

9. Harigaya, S. and Schwartz, A. (1969). Rate of calcium binding and uptake in animal and human cardiac muscle: Membrane vesicles ('relaxing system') and mitochondria. Circ. Res., **25**, 781.

10. Hasselbach, W. and Makinose, M. (1962). ATP and active transport. Biochem. biophys. Res. Com., **7**, 132.

11   Honig, C.R. and Nierop, C. van (1964). The possible relationship between cardiac relaxing substance and cyclic adenosine 3', 5'-monophosphate. Biochim. biophys. acta, **86**, 355.

12   Inesi, G., Ebashi, S. and Watanabe, S. (1964). Preparation of vesicular relaxing factor from bovine heart tissue. Amer. J. Physiol., **207**, 1339.

13   Katz, A.M. (1970). Contractile proteins of the heart. Physiol. Rev., **50**, 63.

14   Katz, A.M. and Hecht, H.A. (1969). The early 'pump' failure of the ischemic heart. Amer. J. Med., **47**, 497.

15   Lee, K.S. (1965). Present status of cardiac relaxing factor. Fed. Proc., **24**, 1432.

16   Luttgau, H.C. (1963). The action of calcium ions on K^+ contractures of single muscle fibers. J. Physiol., **168**, 679.

17   Luttgau, H.C. and Niedergerke, R. (1958). The angatonism between calcium and Na^+ ions on the frog's heart. J. Physiol., **143**, 386.

18   Marsh, B.B. (1951). A factor modifying muscle fibre syneresis. Nature, Lond., **167**, 1065.

19   McCollum, W.B., Crow, C., Harigaya, S., Bajusz, E. and Schwartz, A. (1970). J. mol. cell. Cardiol. (in press).

20   Niedergerke, R. (1963). Movements of calcium in beating ventricles of the frog heart. J. Physiol., **167**, 551.

21   Ohnishi, T. and Ebashi, S. (1963). Spectrophotometric measurement of instantaneous calcium binding of the relaxing factor of muscle. J. Biochem., **54**, 506.

22   Schwartz, A., Allen, J.C. and Harigaya, S. (1969). Possible involvement of cardiac Na^+, K^+-ATPase in the mechanism of action of cardiac glycosides. J. Pharmacol., **168**, 31.

23   Uchida, K. and Mommaerts, W.F.H.M. (1963). Modification of the contractile responses of actomyosin cyclic adenosine 3', 5'-phosphate. Biochem. biophys. Res. Com., **10**, 1.

24 Weber, A. (1966). Energized calcium transport and relaxing factors. In 'Current Topics in Bioenergetics'. Sanadi, D.R. (Ed.), vol. 1, pp. 203-254. Academic Press, New York.

25 Weber, A., Herz, R. and Reiss, I. (1963). On the mechanism of the relaxing effect of fragmented sarcoplasmic reticulum. J. gen. Physiol., **46**, 679.

26 Weber, A., Herz, R. and Reiss, I. (1964). The regulation of myofibrillar activity by calcium. Proc. Roy. Soc., **B160**, 489.

27 Weyne, J. (1966). Actions des ions strontium sur le muscle cardiaque. C.R. Soc. Biol., Paris, **160**, 210.

CALCIUM AND THE MITOCHONDRIA*

W. KÜBLER and E.A. SHINEBOURNE

Abteilung für Kardiologie, Universität Düsseldorf
and Institute of Cardiology, University of London

Calcium-activity within the myocardial cell depends on several factors:

(1) Calcium can be passively bound within the cell. In the ischemic myocardium — when all ATP has been broken down — most of the calcium is bound to the fraction sedimented between 0 and 1000 x g (Fig. 1). Apart from this fraction, the mitochondrial and microsomal fractions, which are spun down at higher g-values, are also capable of passive calcium-binding.

(2) Calcium can be present as an undissociated and thus inactive complex. This condition may be in the myocardium of major importance, as can be seen from the results presented in Fig. 2. The 200,000 x g supernatant of canine myocardial homogenate has been passed through a high-voltage electrical field in a

---

*Some of the experiments mentioned in this paper were supported by a grant from the Deutsche Forschungsgemeinschaft (Germany) or by the Medical Research Council (Great Britain).

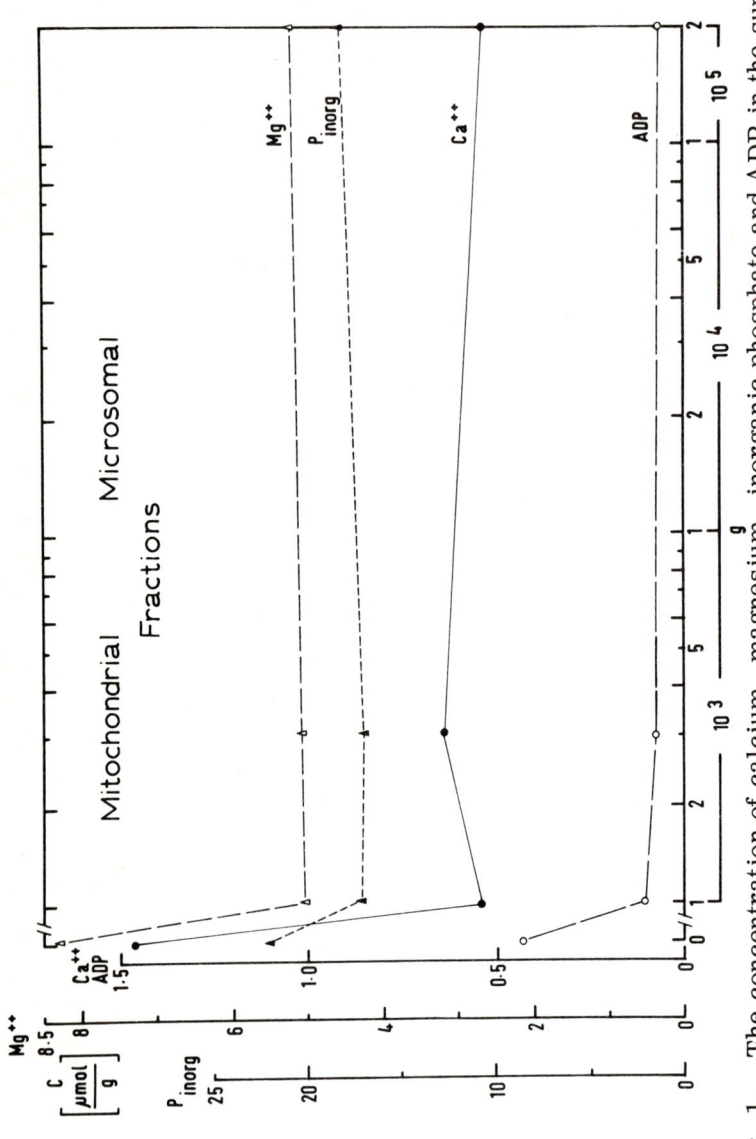

Fig. 1. The concentration of calcium, magnesium, inorganic phosphate and ADP in the supernatant of homogenized canine myocardium after centrifugation at different g-values. Each point is the mean of six experiments.

thin buffer-film. Under these conditions the ions of completely dissociated solutions move towards the anode and cathode to form electrical double layers. Using a myocardial extract, however, an additional peak appears, which is due to undissociated electrically less active complexes, which are not diverted under an electrical field. As can be seen from the results in Fig. 2, at least 50% of the divalent cations present in a myocardial extract are not dissociated, but exact quantitative figures cannot be given.

(3) There is electrophysiological evidence of calcium-exchange across the cardiac cell membrane with an inflow during depolarisation and an outflow during repolarisation.[69]

(4) Calcium can be actively bound — for example to the microsomal membranes in the presence of ATP (Schwartz, this Symposium).

(5) Calcium can be actively taken up into subcellular structures, either into the microsomal or into the mitochondrial fraction. The latter process will be mainly the topic of this paper.

Electro-mechanical coupling which is believed to be due to changes in the myocardial Ca^{++} activity must be related to a process fast enough to release and bind enough calcium necessary for contraction during each cardiac cycle. In skeletal muscle it is almost universally accepted that the intracellular calcium movements during relaxation depend on the sarcoplasmic reticulum.[29, 31, 39, 50, 61, 88] In cardiac muscle, however, active calcium accumulation by the sarcoplasmic reticulum is much less than in skeletal muscle, both in the presence[34, 45] and absence of oxalate,[46, 65, 90] the microsomal binding constant for calcium

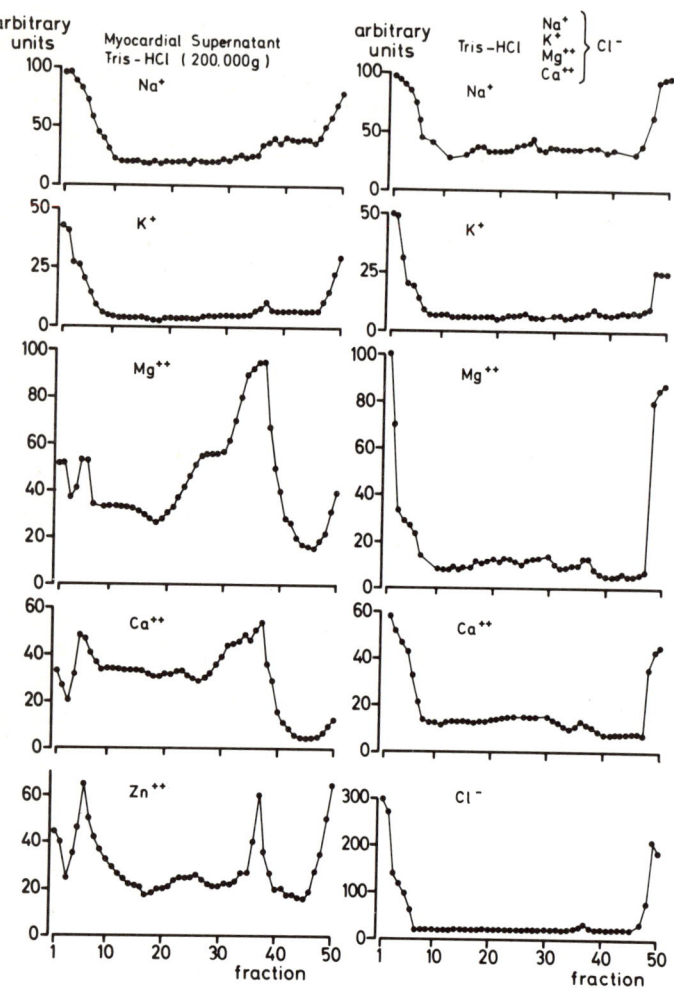

Fig. 2

being in cardiac muscle only about a quarter of that in skeletal muscle.[38,46]

On the other hand, the myocardium contains more mitochondria than does skeletal muscle. Therefore a possible role of the energy-dependent mitochondrial calcium transport system for cardiac contraction-relaxation process has been suggested.[18,40,54,62,89] This conclusion was reached by Patriarca and Carafoli[62] when they found intraperitoneally injected ^{45}calcium to be concentrated in the mitochondria rather than in the microsomal fraction of rat heart. The predominant accumulation of injected ^{45}calcium in myocardial mitochondria does not prove a role of this subcellular structure in contraction-relaxation, as these results do not necessarily show that the mitochondrial calcium is easily exchangeable. It could also be possible that the injected ^{45}calcium was originally taken up by the microsomes and only

---

Fig. 2. The electrophoretic mobility of electrolytes in a highly dissociated solution (right side) and in a myocardial extract (left side).

After centrifugation at 200,000 x g for 1 hr the supernatant of homogenized canine myocardium was passed through a high voltage electrical field in a thin buffer-film (left side). Under the same experimental conditions the electrophoretic mobility of electrolytes of a highly dissociated solution — all cations being in the chloride-form — was examined.

Buffer-film-electrophoresis VAP II (Dr. Bender and Dr. Hobein, Munich/Germany). Buffer in the electrophoresis chamber: Tris (0.08 m)-HCl, pH 7.4, conductance 0.0016 Ω^{-1} cm^{-1}.
Buffer for the electrodes: Tris (0.32 m)-HCl, pH 7.4. Voltage: 2050 V. Current: 135 mA. Temperature: 4° C.

accumulated secondarily by mitochondria during the preparation procedure.

Similar to the results of Patriarca and Carafoli,[62] Fehmers[35] showed that the amount of calcium in mitochondria isolated from the perfused rat heart changed markedly when the calcium concentration of the fluid perfusing the heart was altered. However, these results also do not prove a role of mitochondria in contraction-relaxation.

Horn et al.[43] and Haugaard et al.[41] studied the effect of epinephrine in hearts poisoned with sufficient iodoacetate to inhibit glycolysis. Whereas the initial positive inotropic response to epinephrine was well established, an increased force of contraction was not maintained unless pyruvate was added as a substrate for the tricarboxylic acid cycle. These results were interpreted in terms of indirect support for the view that mitochondrial reactions play a role in myocardial contractility. The results, however, can also be explained by insufficient ATP generation in hearts with blocked glycolytic flux and no substrate for the tricarboxylic acid cycle. Furthermore, iodoacetate is not a specific inhibitor of the glycolytic enzyme glycerine-aldehyde-phosphate-dehydrogenase (GAPDH), but affects all SH- groups.

Calcium can be accumulated by mitochondria via two principal distinct processes: (1) passive binding, and (2) active uptake. In Fig. 3 kinetic plots for passive calcium binding and for active calcium uptake into mitochondria of pig heart are seen. Passive binding is shown in a Scatchard plot,[81] where two straight lines, representing two different binding sites on the

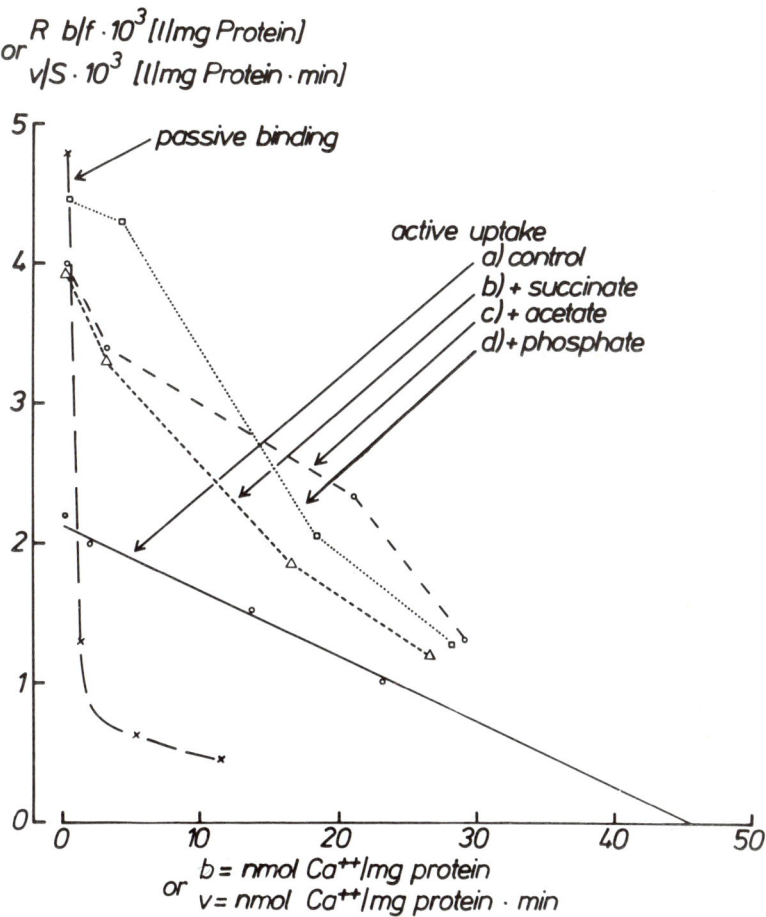

Fig. 3. Passive binding of calcium to pig heart mitochondria shown in a Scatchard-plot (Scatchard[81]) and active calcium uptake by pig heart mitochondria in the absence and present of permeant anions (succinate, acetate and phosphate) shown in an Eadie-Hofstee plot.[28] Each point is the mean of four experiments. In the Scatchard plot two different straight lines can be extrapolated, indicating two different binding sites (see also Fig. 5 from Reynafarje and Lehninger[70]). In the Eadie-Hofstee plot v_{max} is given by the intercept on the abscissa; the intercept on the ordinate represents

(Continued on next page)

mitochondrial membrane, were obtained (see also Fig. 5). Similar to the Scatchard plot for passive binding is the Eadie-Hofstee plot for active uptake.[28] In a graph 'v/S against v (v = velocity, S = substrate concentration)', lines very similar to straight lines were obtained for mitochondrial active calcium uptake with and without permeant anions. The active calcium transport into mitochondria therefore can be described in terms of Michaelis-Menten kinetics in the presence and absence of permeant anions. In the Eadie-Hofstee plot (Fig. 3) v_{max} is given by the intercept of the slope with the abscissa, whilst the intercept on the ordinate represents v_{max}/K_m. Table 1 shows the Michaelis constants (K_m) and maximal velocity (v_{max}) for active calcium uptake into the mitochondria of pig heart. As can be seen, the greatest velocity can be obtained in the assays containing 4 m. molar phosphate as permeant anions, v_{max} being then 45-50 n. mol/mg protein · min and K_m 1 · 10^{-5} m. For a myocardial calcium concentration during contraction of about 10^{-6} m,[87] the velocity of the mitochondrial calcium uptake can be calculated according to the Michaelis-Menten equation: Without permeant anions the velocity

---

Fig. 3 (cont.)

v_{max}/K_m.

Assay conditions: Millipore-filtering technique. ATP: 5 m. mol. $MgCl_2$: 5 m. mol. Temperature: 25° C. Calcium-ion concentrations: 1 · 10^{-7} m and 1 · 10^{-6} m stabilized with EGTA. The calcium concentrations of 9 · 10^{-6} m and 2.2 · 10^{-5} m were calculated using the formation constants for the complexes of ATP with Mg^{++}- or Ca^{++}- ions given by Brunton.[8]

v = 2.1 n. mol/mg protein · min and with phosphate as permeant anion v = 4.3 n. mol/mg protein · min. With the extraction procedure used about 6 mg mitochondrial protein/g myocardium were obtained. According to Langer[51] the relaxation time for cardiac muscle at 20° C and a heart rate of 70-80 beats/minute is not less than 200 m. sec. Therefore the amount of calcium which can be taken up by the mitochondria during the relaxation period would amount in the absence of permeant anions to about 0.04 n. mol/g · 200 m. sec and in the presence of phosphate to 0.09 n. mol/g · 200 m. sec.

For microsomal fractions, Harigaya and Schwartz[38] estimated the rate of energy-dependent microsomal calcium binding to be 4.5-12 n. mol/g · 200 m. sec at room temperature, * that is, about 100 times the amount found for mitochondrial calcium uptake. Based on data of Ebashi et al.,[30] Harigaya and Schwartz[38] estimated the amount of calcium necessary for contraction to be about 60 n. mol/g. The same amount should be removed during relaxation, i.e. 60 n. mol/g · 200 m.sec. That is, about 5-10 times more than the velocity of microsomal calcium binding and approximately 1000 times more than the velocity of mitochondrial calcium uptake.

In order to suggest a possible role of the mitochondria in cardiac contraction-relaxation, it should further be shown that these structures are able to release enough calcium in order to

---

*At this meeting Schwartz reported rates of active calcium binding to the microsomal fraction which are 10 times higher than that previously given.

trigger contraction. Release of calcium from previously loaded mitochondria can be brought on by substrate-free incubation, by incubation in a medium of high potassium or inorganic phosphate concentration or by adding respiratory inhibitors or uncoupling agents to the system.[22, 24] The amount of calcium released is about 100 n. mol/mg protein · 3 min, that equals approximately 0.7 n. mol/g · 200 m. sec. Assuming the same velocity for myocardial contraction as for relaxation, the velocity of calcium-release from the mitochondria is about 100 times too small to account for the release of calcium necessary to trigger contraction.

It must, however, be considered that all these values for mitochondrial calcium movements could be unduly small because of methodological difficulties, i.e. non-optimal assay conditions, poor yield in the preparation of the mitochondria or mitochondrial damage during the preparation procedure.

Although mitochondria can show decreased calcium uptake after only 30 minutes of substrate-free perfusion of the rat heart,[60] the good respiratory control and the reproducible stoichiometric ratios of calcium uptake are arguments against significant damage. Furthermore, most of the preparation procedure is done at 4° C or less. According to morphometric measurements on the arrested canine heart at 5° C (experiments together with Hübner, Spieckermann and Bretschneider) even after four hours of ischemia the mitochondria still contain some granules, loss of which is the first, but fully reversible, morphological sign of ischemic cardiac damage (Fig. 4).[44, 63] Also the high energy phosphates — creatine phosphate (CP) and ATP — indicate that the heart could be adequately resuscitated under these conditions.[47-49]

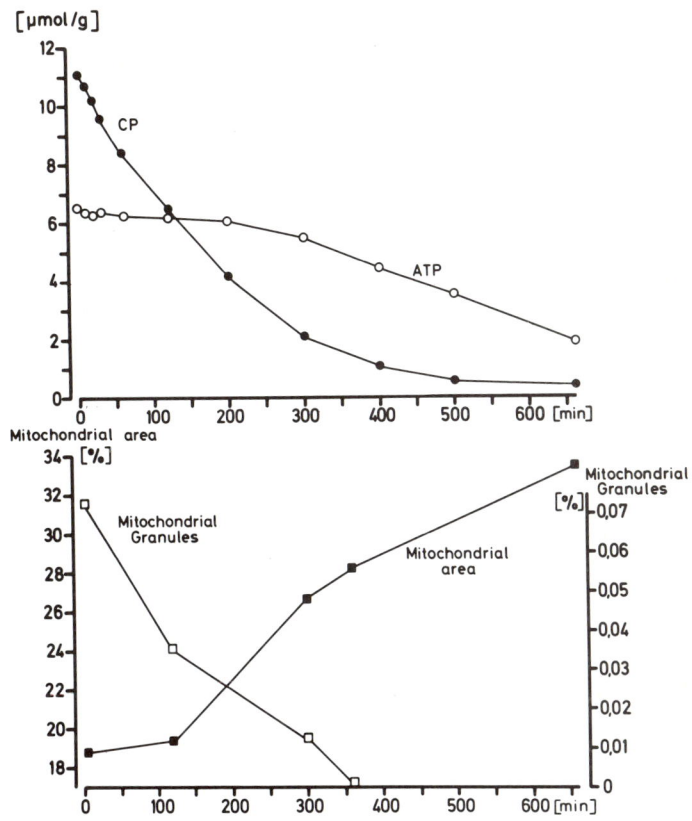

Fig. 4. The breakdown of the high-energy phosphates creatine phosphate (CP) and adenosine triphosphate (ATP) in the ischemic cardioplegic hypothermic (5° C) canine myocardium (upper part of figure). Each point is the mean of 12 experiments. The cardioplegia was done according to Bretschneider[4] and Kübler.[47]

In the lower part of the figure the loss of mitochondrial granules during the ischemic period and the changes in mitochondrial volume of the canine myocardium as determined by morphometry are seen. The experimental conditions were the same as in the experiments of the upper part. Each point is the mean of about 1250 morphometric counts of five different electron microscopic pictures. (Experiments together with Hübner, Spieckermann and Bretschneider.)

Table 1

Maximal velocity (v_{max}) and Michaelis constant (K_m) for active calcium uptake in pig heart mitochondria in the presence and absence of permeant anions. The values were obtained from the results shown in Fig. 3

Ca^{++} uptake by mitochondrial fraction of pig heart, 25° C

Experimental conditions	K_m (µmol)	v_{max} (n. mol/mg protein · min)
Control (no permeant anions)	21	45-50
With succinate (4 m. mol)	12	45-50
With acetate (4 m. mol)	12	45-50
With phosphate (4 m. mol)	10	45-50

As can be seen from the results presented in Fig. 4, in the heart not damaged by anoxia about 20% of the myocardium consists of mitochondria. On a wet weight basis the yield of mitochondria was at least 5 g/100 g myocardium, that is, 25% of the value expected from the morphometric data. However, even if allowance is made for the fact that the yield for the mitochondria is only 25%, the amount of calcium released and taken up by the mitochondrial fraction is still more than 100 times too small to account quantitatively for contraction-relaxation.

In conclusion, there are until now no data available which show calcium uptake and release by myocardial mitochondria to be fast enough to account quantitatively for the contraction-relaxation process. Most of the data were obtained using a millipore-filtering technique; this method is less suitable for recording the initial rate of calcium uptake than the dual-beam spectrophotometry technique with murexide as an indicator of the free calcium ion concentration. The data published by Harigaya and Schwartz[38] and Mela[57] using this method, however, agree well or are at least in the same order of magnitude as those obtained with the millipore-filter technique.

Most of the experiments into the mechanism of passive calcium binding and active calcium uptake were done with liver mitochondria, which are probably in some respects different from cardiac mitochondria, e.g., rat liver mitochondria show no accumulation of magnesium when tested under the same conditions effective in heart mitochondria.[14,64] Therefore the mechanisms of passive calcium binding and active uptake by the mitochondrial fraction will be only briefly discussed. (For further details see Chance[17] and others.[23, 33, 37, 40, 54, 76, 85])

Calcium accumulation by isolated mitochondria can occur either in the absence of energy, by passive binding, or by an active uptake which requires coupled respiration or the hydrolysis of ATP.[54]

Respiratory-inhibited liver mitochondria possess two major classes of energy-independent calcium-binding sites, those of so-called low and high affinity.[70] The two different binding sites are seen in a Scatchard plot[81] (Fig.5; see also Fig. 3), where two straight lines were obtained. About 40 n. mol calcium/mg mitochondrial protein can be bound to the low affinity sites, which are probably identical with the metabolism-independent binding sites described by Rossi et al.,[71] and which can be inhibited by local anaesthetics.[56, 57, 79] According to Scarpa and Azzone[80] the low affinity sites consist of phospholipids; low affinity calcium binding, however, is absent from blowfly muscle mitochondria, which are rich in phosphatidylethanolamine.[12]

The high affinity energy independent binding sites probably represent carrier molecules specific for calcium transport across the mitochondrial membrane.[70] Mela[55, 56] and Mela and Chance[59] showed that lanthanides inhibit specifically energy-dependent calcium uptake into rat liver mitochondria. As the inhibition is non-competitive and the lanthanides concentration necessary for total inhibition of active calcium accumulation is 0.05-0.07 n. mol/mg protein,[57] the number of calcium-specific carrier molecules in the mitochondrial membrane must be less than 0.1

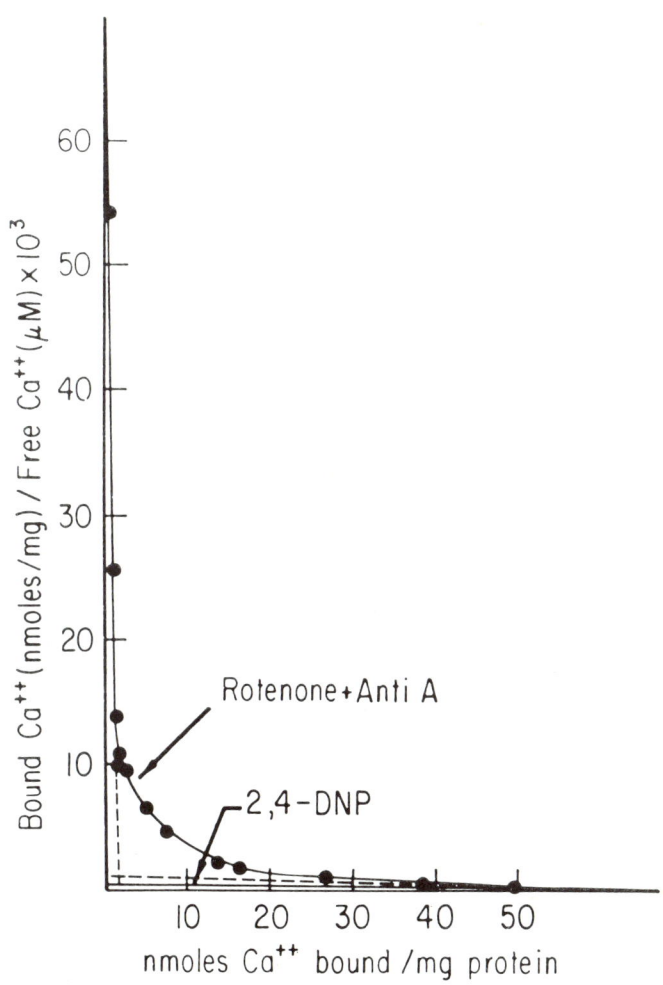

Fig. 5. Scatchard plots [81] of Ca^{++} binding in the presence of respiratory inhibitors and of 2,4-dinitrophenol. No high affinity binding of Ca^{++} took place in the presence of 2,4-dinitrophenol. (From Reynafarje and Lehninger.[70])

n. mol/mg protein. This value is much less than that previously reported by Reynafarje and Lehninger[70] of 1.2 n. mol/mg protein and by Lehninger[52] of 0.6 n. mol/mg protein. Lehninger and Carafoli[53] could not detect the high affinity site of calcium binding in rat heart mitochondria, but this is probably due to the use of the less sensitive [45] calcium method. With the lanthanide-titration technique the calcium carrier could be demonstrated in pigeon heart mitochondria.[59]

This carrier is specifically activated by the divalent cations Ca^{++}, Mn^{++} and Sr^{++} [9-11, 16, 20, 57] but not by the monovalent cations and not by Mg^{++} whose transport across the mitochondrial membrane follows another pathway.[5, 6, 67]

The energy-linked uptake of calcium into mitochondria requires either coupled respiration or hydrolysis of added ATP. When ATP is the energy-source the active calcium transport is inhibited by oligomycin or azide and unaffected by respiratory chain inhibitors. When the energy, however, is provided by oxidative phosphorylation the process is inhibited by respiratory chain inhibitors such as antimycin A or rotenone. The respiratory coupled and the ATP-dependent calcium uptake are both blocked by 2, 4-dinitrophenol. Since oligomycin does not inhibit calcium uptake coupled to oxidative phosphorylation, Brierley et al.[7] as well as Rossi and Lehninger[73] concluded that calcium accumulation is dependent on a hypothetical high-energy intermediate of the respiratory chain that is generated between the respiratory chain and the site of action of oligomycin. This high-energy intermediate would be inhibited by 2, 4-dinitrophenol. Water-washed mitochondria, which have completely lost their ability to form ATP, are still capable of active calcium transport.[86] This favours the conclusion that energy linked mitochondrial calcium uptake depends on a high-energy intermediary of the respiratory chain.

The amount of calcium accumulated is stoichiometric with electron transport or with ATP-hydrolysis if calcium accumulation is accompanied by the uptake of a permeant anion such as phosphate or acetate.[3, 13, 21, 36, 54, 72-74] However, in the absence of permeant anions — e.g. in the presence of chloride — the quantitative relationship between calcium accumulation and electron transport may vary greatly.[13, 54, 72]

In the presence of permeant anions such as acetate, phosphate[20, 74] or even adenine-nucleotides,[15] active calcium transport into the mitochondria is accompanied by an uptake of the anion in the direction of the electrochemical gradient. Electroneutrality during calcium accumulation can be achieved not only by anion uptake but also by ejection of monovalent cations — predominantly hydrogen ions[19, 22, 77] or potassium ions.[54] Cation ejection during calcium uptake is of predominant importance if only impermeant anions — such as chloride — are present.[66] The stoichiometric relationship between calcium uptake and anion inflow or cation ejection, however, depends greatly on the experimental conditions.

Using spectrophotometric measurements, Mela and Chance[58] studied the kinetics of reactions associated with mitochondrial calcium uptake. They found the half-time for the oxidation of cytochrome b due to calcium-activated electron transport to be about 30-50 m.sec. The calcium-induced change in the intramitochondrial pH due to the ejection of hydrogen ions is much slower, the half-time for this process being about 20 sec. These data are further evidence that the metabolic processes accompanying active calcium accumulation into mitochondria are slow compared with the relaxation-velocity of cardiac muscle.

Ouabain does not affect calcium uptake into mitochondria, even after damaging the mitochondria with pentobarbital in the unphysiologically high concentration of 6 m.mol.[1,25,27] According to Dransfeld et al.[25,26] calcium accumulation into mitochondria largely depends on the potassium/sodium quotient (Fig. 6). This finding has been used for a possible explanation of the positive inotropic action of digitalis, which can decrease the intracellular potassium concentration and increase the sodium concentration by inhibiting the sodium-potassium pump. In this way the drug could decrease the potassium/sodium quotient at the mitochondrial membrane, diminish mitochondrial calcium uptake and thus increase the ionised exchangeable sarcoplasmic calcium fraction. However, as changes in the intramyocardial potassium/sodium quotient after digitalis are at best very small and can also be observed in congestive heart failure or after damage to the heart, compartmentation of the monovalent ions in the myocardium is a necessary assumption for this hypothesis (see Dransfeld:[25] Discussion). For the positive inotropic action of digitalis, however, other explanations exist, which are not related to the mitochondrial fraction.[2]

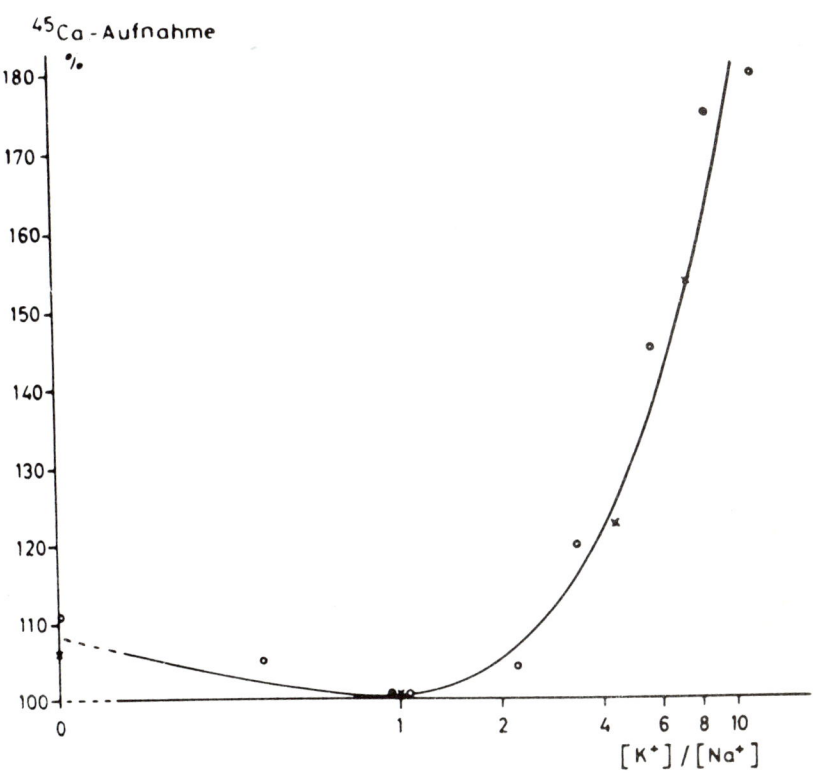

Fig. 6. The influence of the [K⁺]/[Na⁺] quotient in the assay system on Ca⁺⁺ uptake by cardiac mitochondria.
    Experimental conditions:
    Open circles — mitochondria from rabbit heart,
        [K⁺] + [Na⁺] = 130 m. mol.
    Crosses — mitochondria from rabbit heart,
        [K⁺] + [Na⁺] = 90 m. mol.
    Heavy dots — mitochondria from cattle heart,
        [K⁺] + [Na⁺] = 90 m. mol.
(From Dransfeld[25].)

The effects of pharmacological agents on calcium accumulation by mitochondria are very small compared to those on calcium uptake by the sarcoplasmic reticulum. As has been shown previously, noradrenaline[82] and cyclic 3'5'-AMP[32, 83] increase active calcium uptake by microsomes in the presence of oxalate, although calcium accumulation by mitochondria is not significantly affected by these drugs under these conditions (Table 2). Furthermore, drugs such as propranolol and quinidine[42, 78, 84, 91] which suppress microsomal calcium uptake are again without significant effect on mitochondrial calcium accumulation (Table 2).

An inhibition of calcium uptake by the microsomal fraction can also be achieved by urea in concentrations which may well be reached in patients (Fig. 7). The mitochondrial calcium uptake, however, is again not affected by urea. The results show calcium uptake by the microsomes being increased or decreased by the action of different drugs, whereas the mitochondrial calcium uptake seems to be comparatively inert.

Most of the experimental data indicate that mitochondrial calcium uptake and release are not directly related to the contraction-relaxation process in the heart. As one of the factors regulating the calcium concentration in the cytoplasmic space, however, the mitochondria could be of importance for determining the amount of calcium available for the contraction-relaxation process. In this way myocardial contractility could indirectly also be related to mitochondrial calcium accumulation. The action of the positive and negative inotropic agents listed in Table 2 could be explained on the basis of a concurrence between mitochondrial and microsomal calcium uptake in the myocardial cell.

Table 2

Changes in active calcium uptake into the microsomal and mitochondrial fraction of pig heart under different conditions. The drugs were given in a concentration of 1 m.mol urea in a concentration of 500 mg %. Failing pig hearts were produced by banding of the pulmonary artery. Each point is the mean of 4-7 experiments.

Experimental conditions	Mitochondrial fraction		Microsomal fraction	
	Change (%)	Significance	Change (%)	Significance
Noradrenaline (1 m.mol)	- 2%	p > 0.1	+33%	p < 0.01
Isoprenaline (1 m.mol)	+27%	p > 0.1	+36%	p < 0.01
3'5'-AMP (1 m.mol)	+15%	p > 0.1	+72%	p < 0.01
Lignocaine (1 m.mol)	+14%	p > 0.1	+ 9%	p > 0.1
Propranolol (1 m.mol)	+13%	p > 0.1	-28%	p < 0.01
Quinidine (1 m.mol)	+16%	p > 0.1	-29%	p < 0.01
Urea (500 mg %)	+10%	p > 0.1	-47%	p < 0.01
Failed heart	-17%	p > 0.1	+35%	

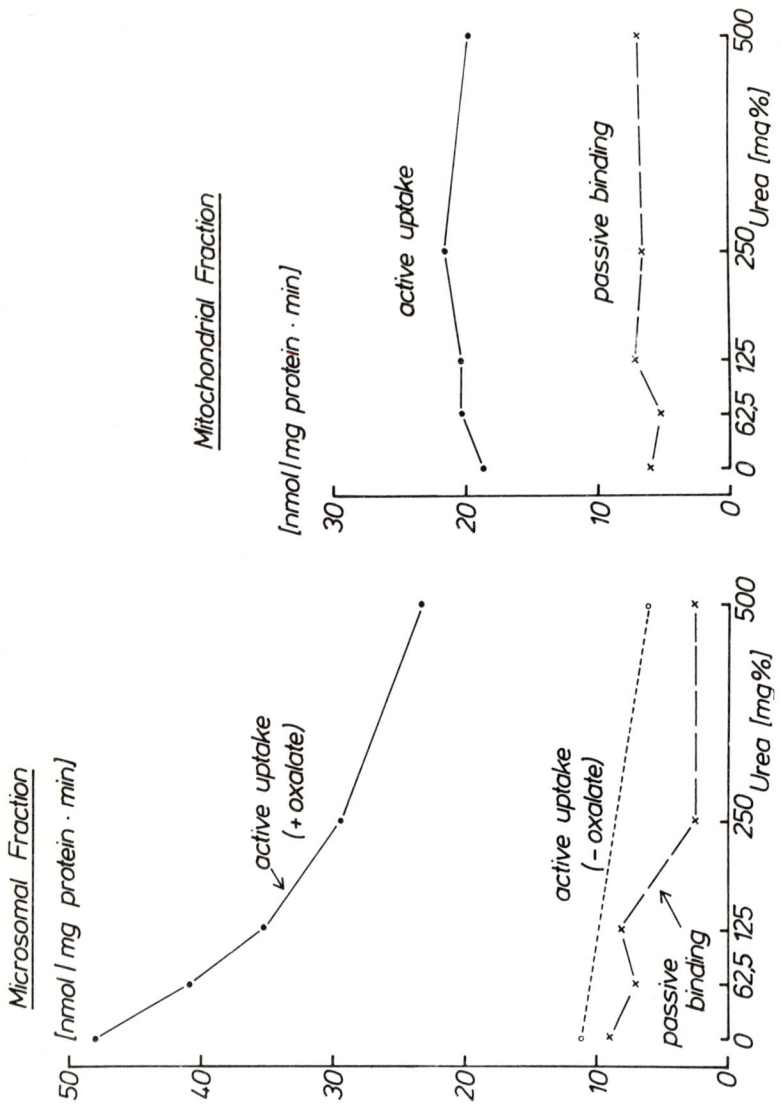

Fig. 7. Passive calcium-binding and active calcium-uptake by microsomal and mitochondrial fractions of pig heart in the presence of different concentrations of urea. Each point is the mean of 3-4 experiments. (Assay conditions: see Fig. 3.)

References

1 Besch, H.R., jr., Allen, J.C., Glick, G. and Schwartz, A. (1970). Correlation between the inotropic action of ouabain and its effects on subcellular enzyme systems from canine myocardium. J. Pharmacol., **171**, 1.

2 Besch, H.R., jr. and Schwartz, A. (1970). On a mechanism of action of digitalis. J. mol. cell. Cardiol., **1**, 195.

3 Bielawski, J. and Lehninger, A.L. (1966). Stoichiometric relationships in mitochondrial accumulation of calcium and phosphate supported by hydrolysis of adenosine triphosphate. J. biol. Chem., **241**, 4316.

4 Bretschneider, H.J. (1964). Überlebens- und Wiederbelebungszeit des Herzens bei Normo- und Hypothermie. Verh. dtsch. Ges. Kreisl.-Forsch., **30**, 11.

5 Brierley, G.P., Bachmann, E. and Green, D.E. (1962). Active transport of inorganic phosphate and magnesium ions by beef heart mitochondria. Proc. nat. Acad. Sci., Wash., **48**, 1928.

6 Brierley, G., Murer, E., Bachmann, E. and Green, D.E. (1963). Studies on ion transport. II. The accumulation of inorganic phosphate and magnesium ions by heart mitochondria. J. biol. Chem., **238**, 3482.

7 Brierley, G.P., Murer, E. and Green, D.E. (1963). Participation of an intermediate of oxidative phosphorylation in ion accumulation by mitochondria. Science, **140**, 60.

8 Brunton, K. (1959). Formation constants for the complexes of adenosine di- or triphosphate with magnesium or calcium ions. Biochem. J., **71**, 388.

9 Caplan, A. and Carafoli, E. (1965). The effect of Sr^{2+} on swelling and ATP-linked contraction of mitochondria. Biochim. biophys. acta, **104**, 317.

10 Carafoli, E. (1965a). Active accumulation of Sr^{++} by rat liver mitochondria. II. Competition between Ca^{2+} and Sr^{2+}. Biochim. biophys. acta, **97**, 99.

11 Carafoli, E. (1965b). Active accumulation of Sr^{2+} by rat liver mitochondria. III. Stimulation of respiration by Sr^{2+} and its stoichiometry. Biochim. biophys. acta, **97**, 107.

12 Carafoli, E. (1969). Calcium ion transport in mitochondria. Biochem. Soc. Agenda Papers, pp. 2-3, November.

13 Carafoli, E., Gamble, R. L., Rossi, C. S. and Lehninger, A. L. (1967). Super-stoichiometric ratios between ion movements and electron transport in rat liver mitochondria. J. biol. Chem., **242**, 1199.

14 Carafoli, E., Rossi, C. S. and Lehninger, A. L. (1964). Cation and anion balance during active accumulation of Ca^{++} and Mg^{++} by isolated mitochondria. J. biol. Chem., **239**, 3055.

15 Carafoli, E., Rossi, C. S. and Lehninger, A. L. (1965). Uptake of adenine nucleotides by respiring mitochondria during active accumulation of Ca^{++} and phosphate. J. biol. Chem., **240**, 2254.

16 Carafoli, E., Weiland, S. and Lehninger, A. L. (1965) Active accumulation of Sr^{2+} by rat liver mitochondria. Biochim. biophys. acta, **97**, 88.

17 Chance, B. (1963). (Ed.) 'Energy Linked Functions of Mitochondria'. Academic Press, New York and London.

18 Chance, B. (1964). The energy-linked reaction of calcium with mitochondria. J. biol. Chem., **240**, 2729.

19 Chapell, J. B. and Crofts, A. R. (1965). Calcium ion accumulation and volume changes of isolated liver mitochondria. Biochem. J., **95**, 378.

20 Chapell, J. B. and Greville, G. D. (1963). Isolated mitochondria and accumulation of divalent metal ions. Fed. Proc., **22**, 526.

21 Christianson, R.O., Loyter, A., Steensland, H., Saltzgaber, J. and Racker, E. (1969). Energy-linked ion translocation in submitochondrial particles. II. Properties of submitochondrial particles capable of Ca^{++}-translocation. J. biol. Chem., **244**, 4428.

22 Drahota, Z., Carafoli, E., Rossi, C.S., Gamble, R.L. and Lehninger, A.L. (1965). The steady state maintenance of accumulated Ca^{++} in rat liver mitochondria. J. biol. Chem., **240**, 2712.

23 Drahota, Z. and Ernster, L. (1969). (Eds.) 'Mitochondria, Structure and Function', FEBS Symposium, Vol. 17, Academic Press, London and New York.

24 Drahota, Z. and Lehninger, A.L. (1965). Movements of H^+, K^+ and Na^+ during energy-dependent uptake and retention of Ca^{++} in rat liver mitochondria. Biochem. biophys. Res. Com., **19**, 351.

25 Dransfeld, H. (1968). Zur Wirkung der Digitalisglykoside auf den intrazellulären Elektrolytstoffwechsel. In 'Herzinsuffizienz, Pathophysiologie und Klinik', pp. 549-552. Reindell, H., Keul, J. and Doll, E. (Eds.). Georg Thieme Verlag, Stuttgart.

26 Dransfeld, H., Greeff, K., Hess, D. and Schorn, A. (1967). Die Abhängigkeit der Ca^{++}- Aufnahme isolierter Mitochondrien des Herzmuskels von der $Na^+ + K^+$-Konzentration als mögliche Ursache der inotropen Digitaliswirkung. Experientia, **23**, 375.

27 Dransfeld, H., Greeff, K., Schorn, A. and Ting, B.T. (1969). Calcium uptake in mitochondria and vesicles of heart and skeletal muscle in presence of potassium, sodium k-strophanthin and pentobarbital. Biochem. Pharmacol., **18**, 1335.

28 Eadie, G.S. (1952). On the evaluation of the constants V_m and K_m in enzyme reactions. Science, **116**, 688.

29 Ebashi, S. (1961). Calcium binding activity of vesicular relaxing factors. J. Biochem., **50**, 236.

30 Ebashi, S., Kodama, A. and Ebashi, F. (1968). Troponin: I. Preparation and physiological function. J. Biochem., **64**, 465.

31 Ebashi, S. and Lipmann, F. (1962). Adenosine triphosphate-linked concentrations of calcium ions in a particulate fraction of rabbit muscle. J. Cell Biol., **14**, 389.

32 Entman, M. L., Levy, G. S. and Epstein, S. E. (1969). Mechanism of action of epinephrine and glucagon on the canine heart. Evidence for increase in sarcotubular calcium stores mediated by cyclic 3'5'-AMP. Circ. Res., **25**, 429.

33 Ernster, L. and Lee, C.-P. (1964). Biological oxidoreductions. Ann. Rev. Biochem., **33**, 729.

34 Fanburg, B., Finkel, R. M. and Martonosi, A. (1964). The role of calcium in the mechanism of relaxation of cardiac muscle. J. biol. Chem., **239**, 2298.

35 Fehmers, M. C. O. (1968). Intracellulair Ca^{2+} en de werking van hartspier. Ph. D. Dissertation, University of Amsterdam.

36 Gear, A. R. L., Rossi, C. S., Reynafarje, B. and Lehninger, A. L. (1967). Acid-base exchanges in mitochondria and suspending medium during respiration-linked accumulation of bivalent cations. J. biol. Chem., **242**, 3403.

37 Green, D. E. and Baum, H. (1970). 'Energy and the Mitochondrion'. Academic Press, New York & London.

38 Harigaya, S. and Schwartz, A. (1969). Rate of calcium binding and uptake in normal animal and failing human cardiac muscle. Circ. Res., **25**, 781.

39 Hasselbach, W. and Makinose, M. (1961). Die Calciumpumpe der Erschlaffungsgrana des Muskels und ihre Abhängigkeit von der ATP-Spaltung. Biochem. Z., **333**, 518.

40 Haugaard, N., Haugaard, E. S., Lee, N. H. and Horn, R. S. (1969). Possible role of mitochondria in regulation of cardiac contractility. Fed. Proc., **28**, 1657.

41 Haugaard, N., Lee, N. H., Kostrzewa, R., Horn, R. S. and Haugaard, E. S. (1969). The role of sulfhydril groups in oxidative phosphorylation and ion transport by rat liver mitochondria. Biochim. biophys. acta, **172**, 198.

42 Hess, M. L., Briggs, F. N., Shinebourne, E. and Hamer, J. (1968). Effect of adrenergic blocking agents on the calcium pump of the fragmented cardiac sarcoplasmic reticulum. Nature, Lond., **220**, 79.

43 Horn, R. S., Aronson, C. E., Hess, M. L. and Haugaard, N. N. (1967). The effect of metabolic inhibitors on the response of the perfused rat heart to epinephrine. Biochem. Pharmacol., **16**, 2109.

44 Hübner, G., Paulussen, F., Bretschneider, H. J. and Spieckermann, P. G. (1968). Die Feinstruktur des Herzmuskels bei exakt definierten Funktions- und Stoffwechselbedingungen. Abstr. Fourth European Regional Conference on Electron Microscopy, Rome, p. 307.

45 Inesi, G., Ebashi, S. and Watanabe, S. (1964). Preparation of vesicular relaxing factor from bovine heart tissue. Amer. J. Physiol., **207**, 1339.

46 Katz, A. M. and Repke, D. I. (1967). Quantitative aspects of dog cardiac microsomal calcium binding and calcium uptake. Circ. Res., **21**, 153.

47 Kübler, W. (1967). Nutzbare Ischämiedauer des Herzens in Abhängigkeit von der energetischen Ausgangslage des Myokards, der Kardioplegieform und der Temperatur. Langenbecks Arch. klin. Chir., **319**, 648.

48 Kübler, W. (1969a). Grenzen der Wiederbelebung nach physiologischen und biochemischen Kriterien. Dtsch. med. Wschr., **94**, 1157.

49 Kübler, W. (1969b). Tierexperimentelle Untersuchungen zum Myokardstoffwechsel im Angina-pectoris-Anfall und beim Herzinfarkt. Bibliotheca Cardiologica No. 22. Karger, Basel & New York.

50 Kumagai, H., Ebashi, S. and Takeda, F. (1955). Essential relaxing factor in muscle other than myokinase and creatine phosphokinase. Nature, Lond., **176**, 166.

51 Langer, G. A. (1968). Ion fluxes in cardiac excitation and contraction and their relation to myocardial contractility. Physiol. Rev., **48**, 708.

52 Lehninger, A. L. (1969). Acid-base changes in mitochondria and medium during energy-dependent and energy-independent binding of Ca^{++}. Ann. N. Y. Acad. Sci., **147**, 816.

53 Lehninger, A. L. and Carafoli, E. (1969). In 'Symposium on Control Mechanisms in Intermediary Metabolism'. University of Miami. (From Carafoli, E., 1969.)

54 Lehninger, A. L., Carafoli, E. and Rossi, C. S. (1967). Energy-linked ion movements in mitochondrial systems. Advanc. Enzymol., **29**, 259.

55 Mela, L. (1968a). La^{+++} as a specific inhibitor of divalent cation-induced mitochondrial electron transfer. Fed. Proc., **27**, 828.

56 Mela, L. (1968b). Interactions of La^{+++} and local anesthetic drugs with mitochondrial Ca^{++} and Mn^{++} uptake. Arch. Biochem. Biophys., **123**, 286.

57 Mela, L. (1969). Inhibition and activation of calcium transport in mitochondria. Effects of lanthanides and local anesthetic drugs. Biochemistry, **8**, 2481.

58 Mela, L. and Chance, B. (1968). Spectrophotometric measurements of the kinetics of Ca^{2+} and Mn^{2+} accumulation in mitochondria. Biochemistry, **7**, 4059.

59 Mela, L. and Chance, B. (1969). Calcium carrier and the 'high affinity calcium binding site' in mitochondria. Biochem. biophys. Res. Com., **35**, 556.

60 Muir, J. R., Dhalla, N. S., Orteza, J. M. and Olson, R. E. (1970). Energy-linked calcium transport in subcellular fractions of the failing rat heart. Circ. Res., **26**, 429.

61 Nagai, T., Makinose, M. and Hasselbach, W. (1960). Der physiologische Erschlaffungsfaktor und die Muskelgrana. Biochim. biophys. acta, **43**, 223.

62 Patriarca, P. and Carafoli, E. (1968). A study of the intracellular transport of calcium in rat heart. J. cell. Physiol., **72**, 29.

63 Paulussen, F., Hübner, G., Grebe, D. and Bretschneider, H.J. (1968). Die Feinstruktur des Herzmuskels während einer Ischämie mit Senkung des Energiebedarfes durch spezielle Kardioplegie. Klin. Wschr., **46**, 165.

64 Pressman, B.C. and Park, J.K. (1963). Competition between magnesium and guanidine for mitochondrial binding sites. Biochem. biophys. Res. Com., **11**, 182.

65 Pretorius, P.J., Pohl, W.G., Smithen, C.S. and Inesi, G. (1969). Structural and functional characterization of dog heart microsomes. Circ. Res., **25**, 487.

66 Rasmussen, H., Chance, B. and Ogata, E. (1965). A mechanism for the reactions of calcium with mitochondria. Proc. nat. Acad. Sci., Wash., **53**, 1069.

67 Rasmussen, H. and Ogata, E. (1966). Parathyroid hormone and the reactions of mitochondria to cations. Biochemistry, **5**, 733.

68 Rasmussen, H., Sallis, J., Fang, M., DeLuca, H.F. and Young, R. (1964). Parathyroid hormone and anion uptake in isolated mitochondria. Endocrinology, **74**, 388.

69 Reuter, H. and Scholz, H. (1968). Der Einfluss von Membranpotentialänderungen und Calcium auf die Aktivierung der Kontraktion isolierter Herzpräparate. In 'Herzinsuffizienz, Pathophysiologie und Klinik'. Reindell, H., Keul, J. and Doll, E. (Eds.), pp. 94-97. Georg Thieme Verlag, Stuttgart.

70 Reynafarje, B. and Lehninger, A.L. (1969). High affinity and low affinity binding of Ca^{++} by rat liver mitochondria. J. biol. Chem., **244**, 584.

71 Rossi, C., Azzi, A. and Azzone, G.F. (1967). Ion transport in liver mitochondria. I. Metabolism-independent Ca^{++}-binding and H^+-release. J. biol. Chem., **242**, 951.

72 Rossi, C. and Azzone, G.F. (1965). H^+/O ratio during Ca^{2+} uptake in rat-liver mitochondria. Biochim. biophys. acta, **110**, 434.

73 Rossi, C.S. and Lehninger, A.L. (1963). Stoichiometric relationships between accumulation of ions by mitochondria and the energy coupling sites in the respiratory chain. Biochem. Z., **338**, 698.

74 Rossi, C.S. and Lehninger, A.L. (1964). Stoichiometry of respiratory stimulation, accumulation of Ca^{++} and phosphate and oxidative phosphorylation in rat liver mitochondria. J. biol. Chem., **239**, 3971.

75 Sallis, J.D., DeLuca, H.F. and Rasmussen, H. (1963). Parathyroid hormone-dependent uptake of inorganic phosphate by mitochondria. J. biol. Chem., **238**, 4098.

76 Sanadi, D.R. (1965). Energy-linked reactions in mitochondria. Ann. Rev. Biochem., **34**, 21.

77 Saris, N.E. (1963). Soc. Sci. Fennica, Commentationes Biol., **28**, 1. (From Lehninger, Carafoli and Rossi, 1967.)

78 Scales, B. and McIntosh, D.A.D. (1968). Effects of propranolol and its optical isomers on the radiocalcium uptake and the adenosine triphosphatases of skeletal and cardiac sarcoplasmic reticulum fractions (SRF). J. Pharmacol., **160**, 261.

79 Scarpa, A. and Azzi, A. (1968). Cation binding to submitochondrial particles. Biochim. biophys. acta, **150**, 473.

80 Scarpa, A. and Azzone, G.F. (1969). Effects of phospholipids in liver mitochondria, osmotic properties and binding of cations. Biochim. biophys. acta, **173**, 78.

81 Scatchard, G. (1949). The attractions of proteins for small molecules and ions. Ann. N.Y. Acad. Sci., **51**, 660.

82 Shinebourne, E.A., Hess, M.L., White, R.J. and Hamer, J. (1969). The effect of noradrenaline on the calcium uptake of the sarcoplasmic reticulum. Cardiovasc. Res., **3**, 113.

83 Shinebourne, E. and White, R. (1970). Cyclic AMP and calcium uptake of the sarcoplasmic reticulum in relation to increased rate of relaxation under the influence of catecholamines. Cardiovasc. Res., **4**, 194.

84 Shinebourne, E., White, R. and Hamer, J. (1969). A qualitative distinction between the beta blocking and local anaesthetic actions of antiarrhythmic agents. Circ.Res., **24**, 835.

85 Slater, E.C., Kaninga, Z. and Wojtczak, L. (1967). (Eds.) 'Biochemistry of Mitochondria'. Academic Press, New York and London.

86 Vasington, F.D. and Greenawalt, J.W. (1964). Ca^{++} and P_i uptake by non-phosphorylating mitochondrial preparations. Biochem.biophys.Res.Com., **15**, 133.

87 Weber, A. (1966). Energized calcium transport and relaxing factors. Current Topics in Bioenergetics, **1**, 203.

88 Weber, A., Herz, R. and Reiss, I. (1963). On the mechanism of the relaxing effect of fragmented sarcoplasmic reticulum. J.gen.Physiol., **46**, 679.

89 Weber, A., Herz, R. and Reiss, I. (1964). Role of calcium in contraction and relaxation of muscle. Fed.Proc., **23**, 896.

90 Weber, A., Herz, R. and Reiss, I. (1967). Nature of the cardiac relaxing factor. Biochim.biophys.acta, **131**, 188.

91 White, R. and Shinebourne, E. (1969). The interaction of sympathetic stimulation and blockade on the calcium uptake of the sarcoplasmic reticulum. Cardiovasc.Res., **3**, 245.

> **ERRATUM**
>
> The names of Philip and Harriet Goodhart should not appear as co-authors of Arnold M. Katz's paper "Calcium and the Cardiac Contractile Proteins" on Page 124.

CALCIUM AND THE CARDIAC CONTRACTILE PROTEINS*

ARNOLD M. KATZ
and
PHILIP J. and HARRIET L. GOODHART

The Mount Sinai School of Medicine of the City University
of New York, New York City, New York 10029

In this brief presentation I would like to set forth a model that describes the nature of the interaction between calcium ion (Ca^{++}) and the cardiac contractile proteins, and to examine some of the physiological consequences of this model. As will become apparent, major discrepancies exist between the behavior of the cardiac contractile proteins that this model predicts, and many of the measurements reported by workers in the field of cardiac muscle mechanics. Thus, as with any model, its value lies in its drawing into perspective a large body of complex experimentation, rather than defining a

---

*Supported by Research Grants from the U.S. Public Health Service and New York Heart Association. This article, which is based on a Physiological Review written by the author,[7] contains few literature references. Readers wishing to find documentation for many of the observations described herein are referred to this review.

final statement as to the nature of the process described.

At the present time, four named proteins comprise the contractile element of heart muscle: myosin, actin, tropomyosin and troponin (of these, at least one, troponin, consists of more than one discrete protein).

From an experimental viewpoint, calcium has two types of action on these contractile proteins in vitro. The first is that of a direct activator of myosin ATPase activity. This property is seen with highly purified myosin and with actomyosins (actin plus myosin) prepared either with or without the modulatory proteins, tropomyosin and troponin. The property of Ca^{++} to activate myosin ATPase is shared by a number of other cations, with the notable exception of Mg^{++} which inhibits myosin ATPase activity. While striking as an in-vitro phenomenon, the direct activation of myosin ATPase by Ca^{++} probably plays no role in the physiological control of the contractile protein interaction. This is because the depressant action of Mg^{++} on both myosin and actomyosin is predominant and prevents Ca^{++} from stimulating ATPase activity. Such an inhibiting effect is probably present in the living muscle cell in which the contractile proteins are exposed to millimolar concentrations of Mg^{++}. Thus, the addition or deletion of small (micromolar) quantities of calcium would be expected to have no effect on the Mg^{++}-inhibited contractile proteins of the myocardium.

The second action of Ca^{++} upon the cardiac contractile proteins now appears to be directly related to the physiological control of muscular contraction. This action, which is manifest in vitro as a stimulation of the Mg^{++} activated actomyosin ATPase activity,

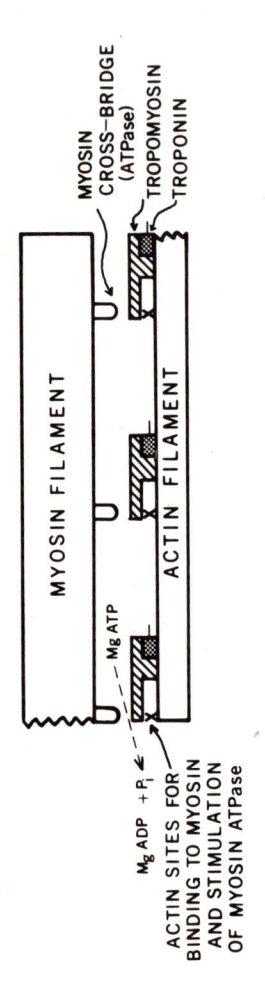

Fig. 1

Fig. 1. Schematic diagram indicating possible interactions between the two contractile proteins, actin and myosin, and the two modulatory proteins, tropomyosin and troponin. Top figure illustrates resting condition (diastole) where, in the absence of Ca^{++}, the modulatory proteins inhibit the interaction between actin and myosin. In this diagram tropomyosin is suggested to be the interaction inhibitor in view of a similar but calcium-independent effect of tropomyosin in the absence of troponin. During systole (lower figure) addition of calcium abolishes inhibition of the actin-myosin interaction by the tropomyosin-troponin complex. Details of these structural changes are unknown, but appear to result from binding of calcium to troponin and an action of troponin and tropomyosin together that requires intact troponin sulfhydryl groups. Release of the inhibitory action of the modulatory proteins permits both the ATPase-stimulating and physicochemical interactions between actin and myosin to proceed, thereby establishing the active state and permitting the muscle to shorten and do work. Maximal shortening velocity of the muscle (v_{max}) appears to be determined by the rate at which the actin-activated myosin cross bridges hydrolyze ATP, and maximum tension (P_o) appears to reflect the number of strong physicochemical interactions between actin and myosin. (Reprinted with permission from Katz.[7])

results from the interaction of Ca^{++} with troponin, one of the modulatory proteins which act upon actin in the thin filament of the sarcomere. Thus, when Ca^{++} is not available to bind to troponin, the interaction between actin and myosin is inhibited so that the Mg^{++}-activated ATPase is low. In vitro, under suitable conditions of ATP and Mg^{++} concentrations and of ionic strength, ATPase is at the low level of that of myosin. Addition of small amounts of Ca^{++} will permit this ion to be bound by troponin A, the component of troponin that has a high-affinity calcium-binding site. As a result of this Ca^{++}-troponin interaction in vitro, the inhibitory action of the troponin-tropomyosin complex is abolished and ATPase becomes activated by actin. In the living muscle, it appears that the Ca^{++}-troponin interaction exposes the myosin-binding sites of the thin (actin) filament, allowing contraction to proceed. Thus this second effect of Ca^{++} upon the contractile proteins, which is apparent in vitro as an activation of actomyosin ATPase activity, does not reflect a direct stimulatory action but, instead, results from a depression of sites on the thin filament. These phenomena have been summarized in the model shown in Fig. 1.

Recent studies of the actions of the troponin complex have added valuable detail to our understanding of the specific reactions involved in this physiological action of Ca^{++}. As has been so often the case, contractile proteins once thought to constitute a single entity have been found to be composed of several discrete proteins. Thus troponin is now recognized to consist of two or more components[3,4] one of which (troponin A) constitutes the calcium-binding protein of the myofibril. More precise knowledge of the interactions of these troponin components can be expected to clarify the biochemical mechanism that permits Ca^{++} to initiate systole by exposing the active sites of the thin filament.

Most studies to date indicate that the calcium-binding site on troponin A can exist in only two states. In the first, when troponin A is devoid of Ca^{++}, the modulatory proteins exert their full inhibitory effect upon the thin filament and contraction is prevented, whereas when Ca^{++} is bound to troponin A, this inhibition is released permitting the muscle to shorten and to generate tension. Thus, variations in the amount of Ca^{++} made available for binding to troponin during excitation-contraction coupling would be expected to modify the number of active sites on the thin filament, but not the properties of the derepressed site, the latter being a reflection of the primary actin-myosin interaction. This biochemical formulation, however, is in direct conflict with a number of observations based upon studies of the mechanical behavior of cardiac muscle.

The biochemical significance of the intercepts of the force-velocity curve of active muscle was explicitly stated by A.V. Hill in his classical 1938 paper.[5] In describing the influence of load on shortening velocity, Hill noted that contracting muscle behaved as if it contained a series of active points which could either be attracted to each other, thereby generating tension, or they could be exposed to take part in chemical reactions during which chemical energy would be liberated at the maximal rate possible for the muscle. If all the active points were attracted to each other, the muscle would not shorten but would, instead, exert its maximal tension (P_o). If, on the other hand, all of the active points were free to participate in chemical reactions, no tension would be exerted and the muscle would shorten at its maximal rate (V_{max}). The maximal rate of shortening thus would depend on the intrinsic properties of the contractile machinery.

The year after Hill published this analysis, the ATPase activity of myosin was discovered. It was not until the middle of the 1960's, however, that a number of investigators noted that the ATPase activity of the myosins from different skeletal muscles were dissimilar, with myosins from the more rapidly contracting muscles having the higher enzymatic activity. The view that myosin ATPase activity was a reflection of the same time-dependent process that determines V_{max} in a given muscle was confirmed by a number of studies, the most extensive being that of Bárány,[1] who examined the relationship between the mechanical and chemical properties of a number of muscles differing widely in both V_{max} and myosin ATPase. This study clearly demonstrated the close correlation between the ATPase activity of highly purified myosin and the maximal shortening velocity of a muscle, while showing that tension correlated not with this enzymatic activity but, instead, with the amount of actomyosin contained in the muscle. From a biochemical standpoint, therefore, it is reasonable to conclude that V_{max} is a reflection of myosin ATPase activity while P_o is determined by a number of actin-myosin interactions per unit of cross-sectional area (Fig. 2).

Theoretical considerations have also led to the conclusion that the maximal shortening velocity of a muscle is independent of the number of active sites. In formulating his theory of muscle contraction with the assumptions that the rates of reaction by which

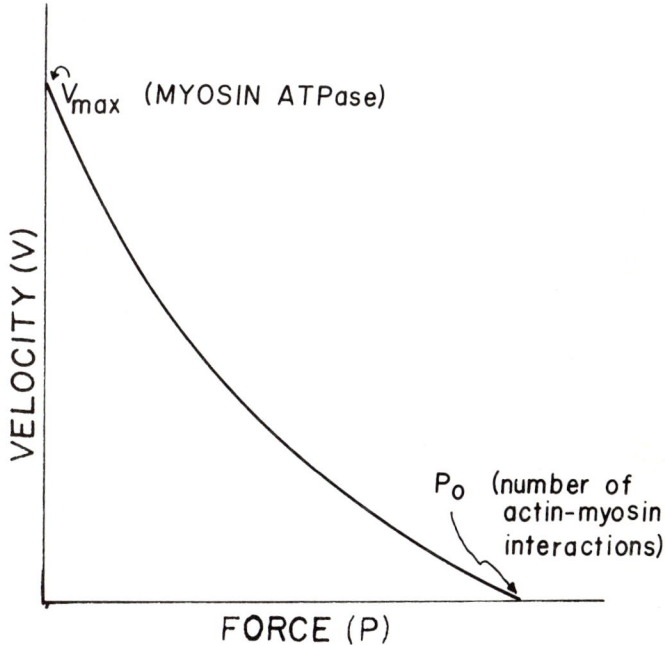

Fig. 2. Schematic drawing of a force-velocity curve illustrating the postulated dependence of V_{max} (rate of shortening at zero load) on myosin adenosine triphosphatase (rate of chemical reaction), and of P_o (maximal tension developed) on the number of actin-myosin interactions that generate tension.

connections between thick and thin filaments are made or broken depend on the relative positions of interacting sites and the intrinsic properties of these sites, A. F. Huxley[6] noted that the speed of unloaded shortening should be independent of the degree of activation. More recently, Katz[7], on reviewing the current biochemical evidence relating to the action of Ca^{++} in effecting excitation-contraction coupling, concluded that the final step in excitation-contraction coupling reflected control by means of the reversible interaction of Ca^{++} with troponin. If this latter view is correct, the contractile proteins can have only two possible physiological states. During relaxation there would be complete inactivation of the binding sites of the thin filament by the troponin-tropomyosin complex, whereas during contraction the binding of Ca^{++} to troponin would fully reverse this inhibitory effect on the thin filament (Fig. 1). Experimental confirmation of this view has been presented by Teichholz and Podolsky,[9] who found that in the 'skinned' muscle fiber preparation maximal shortening velocity was the same at two levels of Ca^{++} concentration, although maximal force varied up to 4-fold as the availability of Ca^{++} for binding to troponin was altered. These findings lend strong support to the view that the availability of activator (Ca^{++}) does not influence the maximal velocity of unloaded contraction.

Studies of the mechanical properties of cardiac muscle have provided evidence that the maximal velocity of shortening is not constant; but instead, that it changes during the evolution of a single contraction[2] and as the result of a variety of inotropic agents, including extracellular Ca^{++} levels.[8] These observations cannot now be explained by the findings and theories outlined above, because these biochemical and biophysical formulations predict that changes in the amount of activator (Ca^{++}), occurring either during the evolution of a single contraction or as the result of an inotropic intervention, would alter the number of active interactions between actin and myosin without influencing the rate of each active interaction. Thus, changes in the availability of Ca^{++} for binding to the calcium receptor of the contractile proteins should modify P_o, but not V_{max}. We are therefore faced with a major discrepancy which can be explained only if inaccuracies are present: (a) in the biochemical interpretation that excitation-contraction coupling is effected by an 'on-off' mechanism; (b) in the biophysical analyses linking the maximal velocity of unloaded shortening to the intrinsic rate of myosin ATPase; or (c) in the mechanical measurements of the maximal velocity of unloaded shortening. Additional work will be needed to resolve this problem.

References

1. Bárány, M. (1967). ATPase activity of myosin correlated with speed of muscle shortening. J. gen. Physiol., **50**, 197.

2. Edman, K.A. and Nilsson, E. (1968). The mechanical parameters of myocardial contraction studies at a constant length of the contractile element. Acta physiol. scand., **72**, 205.

3. Greaser, M.L. and Gergely, J. (1970). Calcium binding component of troponin. Fed. Proc., **29**, 463 abs.

4. Hartshorne, D.J., Theiner, M. and Mueller, H. (1969). Studies on troponin. Biochim. biophys. acta, **175**, 320.

5. Hill, A.V. (1938). The heat of shortening and the dynamic constants of muscle. Proc. Roy. Soc., ser. B, **126**, 136.

6. Huxley, A.F. (1957). Muscle structure and theories of contraction. Prog. Biophys. Chem., **7**, 257.

7. Katz, A.M. (1970). Contractile proteins of the heart. Physiol. Rev., **50**, 63.

8. Sonnenblick, E.H. (1962). Force velocity relationships in mammalian heart muscle. Amer. J. Physiol., **202**, 931.

9. Teichholz, L.E. and Podolsky, R.J. (1970). Force-velocity relations in skinned fibers. Biophys. Soc. Abs., **10**, 218a.

SPECIFIC INHIBITORS AND PROMOTERS OF CALCIUM ACTION IN THE EXCITATION-CONTRACTION COUPLING OF HEART MUSCLE AND THEIR ROLE IN THE PREVENTION OR PRODUCTION OF MYOCARDIAL LESIONS

A. FLECKENSTEIN

Physiological Institute, University of Freiburg, Germany

Excitation occurs at the cardiac fibre membrane whereas contraction is an intracellular phenomenon. Therefore, so that the internal mechanical reactions can be linked with the superficial excitation process, there must be some kind of information transfer from the fibre surface to the intracellular contractile elements. Nature has solved this difficult problem by using Ca ions as a transmitter substance. It is well established that an increased transmembrane Ca influx takes place during excitation together with a liberation of Ca from certain endoplasmic stores probably situated in the longitudinal tubular system. There is overwhelming evidence that this rapid increase in the intracellular concentration of free Ca ions during excitation initiates the splitting of ATP by the Ca-dependent ATPase

---

*The present work was reported at the Meeting of the European Section of the International Study Group for Research in Cardiac Metabolism in London on 6th September, 1970.

of the myofibrils so that phosphate bond energy is transformed into mechanical work. Thus the Ca ions act as mediators between the bioelectrical events at the surface and the intracellular biochemical processes which utilize ATP for contraction. Accordingly, the mechanical activity of the excited myocardium can be completely abolished by removal of Ca without a major impairment of the excitatory processes.

Fig. 1 shows a fundamental experiment in which an electrically stimulated rabbit papillary muscle was put into a Ca-free Tyrode solution. Single fibre action potentials and isometric mechanograms were continuously recorded. As expected, isometric peak tension falls to almost zero within 14 minutes in the Ca-free environment whereas the action potentials do not appreciably change. So, after the loss of mechanical responses, the Ca-deficient myocardium behaves like a nerve where only bioelectrical excitation waves are conducted. However, the mechanical function of the cardiac fibres can be rapidly restored on return to a normal Ca-containing medium. Biochemically, the Ca-deficient myocardium exhibits a striking inability to split its high-energy phosphate compounds during the state of excitation. But after addition of Ca the high-energy phosphate utilization returns to normal.[10, 15, 16, 18, 49] If, on the other hand, the extracellular Ca concentration is increased above normal, more Ca is taken up by the beating heart so that both splitting of high-energy phosphates and contractility are potentiated.

All these observations clearly show that Ca ions not only trigger the contractile process but also control quantitatively the output

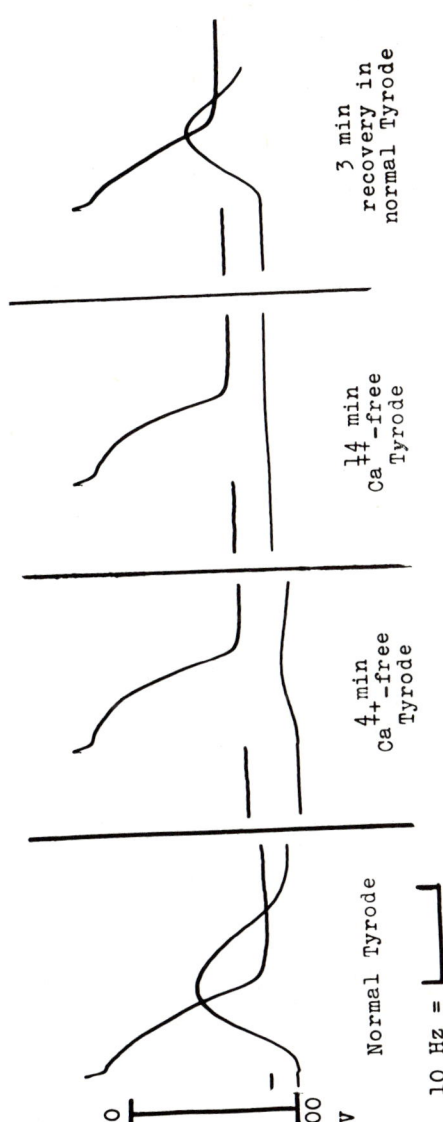

Fig. 1. Complete loss of contractility of an isolated rabbit papillary muscle in a Ca-free Tyrode solution at 37° C. Rapid recovery in ordinary Tyrode solution. Rate of stimulation: 3 shocks/min. Potentials were measured with intracellular microelectrodes of conventional type. Isometric tensions were recorded with a transducer valve (RCA 5734).

of mechanical tension by regulating the amount of ATP which is metabolized during activity. These findings on intact myocardial fibres agree with the results obtained on subcellular muscle constituents, e.g. isolated myofibrils or contractile proteins, which were also found to require the addition of Ca for superprecipitation and maximal ATP-ase activity (for references, see Katz[33]). It should be noted further that a Ca-dependent splitting of ATP also seems to take place during relaxation which is probably initiated by the removal of free Ca ions from the myofibrils by an active transport system. This concentrates Ca in the vesicular components of the sarcoplasmic reticulum by means of an ATP-driven Ca-pump.[8, 9, 25]

I. INHIBITORS OF EXCITATION-CONTRACTION COUPLING

The key role of Ca in excitation-contraction coupling becomes even more evident by virtue of the fact that many substances produce a positive or negative inotropic effect by enhancing the Ca action on utilization of high-energy phosphates or by interfering with it. Bivalent cobalt or nickel ions, for instance, compete with the Ca ions in such a way that excitation-contraction coupling can be abolished as is the case in complete Ca deficiency. Thus, as shown in Fig. 2, a selective loss of contractility is produced on guinea-pig papillary muscles by the addition of 2 mM $NiCl_2$ or $CoCl_2$ to one litre of a normal Tyrode solution containing 1.8 mM $CaCl_2$. But if more $CaCl_2$ is administered the influence of the Co and Ni ions is rapidly overcome, and the original strength of contraction returns to normal. However, the height and the shape of

Table 1

Specific Ca-antagonistic inhibitors of excitation-contraction coupling of mammalian myocardium.

Compound	Structure
Prenylamine (Segontin) Farbwerke Hoechst	(C₆H₅)₂CH—CH₂—CH₂—NH—CH(CH₃)—CH₂—C₆H₅
Verapamil (Isoptin, Iproveratril) Knoll AG Ludwigshafen	(CH₃O)₂C₆H₃—C(CH(CH₃)₂)(C≡N)—CH₂—CH₂—CH₂—N(CH₃)—CH₂—CH₂—C₆H₃(OCH₃)₂
Compound D 600 Knoll AG Ludwigshafen	(CH₃O)₃C₆H₂—C(CH(CH₃)₂)(C≡N)—CH₂—CH₂—CH₂—N(CH₃)—CH₂—CH₂—C₆H₃(OCH₃)₂
Compound Bay a 1040 Bayer-Werke Elberfeld	Formula not yet officially disclosed

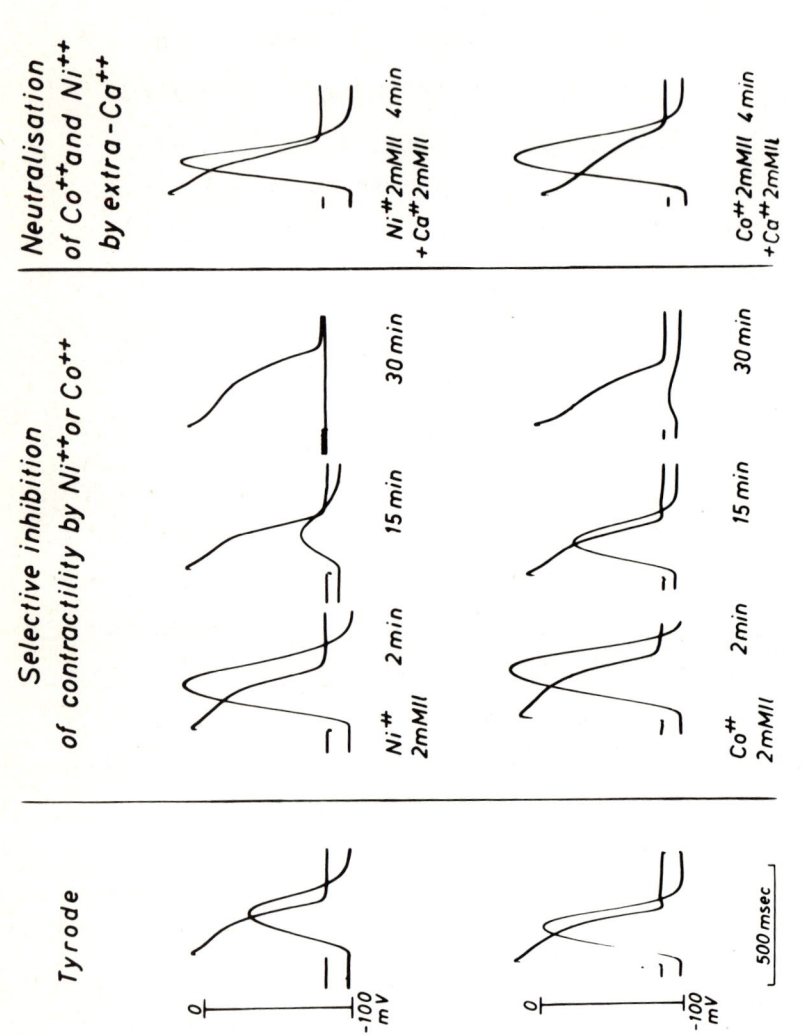

Fig. 2

the action potential do not change appreciably during the whole experiment. This Co-induced contractile failure of the myocardium was first described by Kaufmann and Fleckenstein.[34] One year later, in Canada, a chronic form of Co-induced heart incompetence was found by Sullivan et al.[54] in heavy beer drinkers since some breweries had added $CoCl_2$ to the beer in order to improve the foam.[26]

In an extensive search for other substances which might also be capable of lowering contractile tension of the heart by inhibiting excitation-contraction coupling we have found during the last seven years more than 30 drugs with clear Ca-antagonistic side-effects. These substances include a certain number of adrenergic β-receptor blocking compounds, antifibrillatory drugs, barbituric acid derivatives, and some local anesthetics.[18]

Much more interesting, however, has been the discovery of a new group of extremely potent Ca antagonists (Table I) which can inhibit excitation-contraction coupling in a highly specific way, probably by blocking special Ca channels in the mammalian cardiac muscle fibre membranes. The first reports about the pronounced negative-inotropic effects of these drugs were published by

---

Fig. 2. Isolated guinea-pig papillary muscles lose their contractility within 30 min after addition of 2 mM/l. $NiCl_2$ or $CoCl_2$ to a normal Tyrode solution containing 1.8 mM Ca/l., whereas the single fibre action potentials persist. The effects of Co and Ni can be rapidly neutralized by an extra dose of 2 mM $CaCl_2$/l., so that contractility recovers within 4 min. Rate of stimulation: 30 shocks/min. Temperature: 33° C. Methods as in Fig. 1. (From Kaufmann and Fleckenstein.[34])

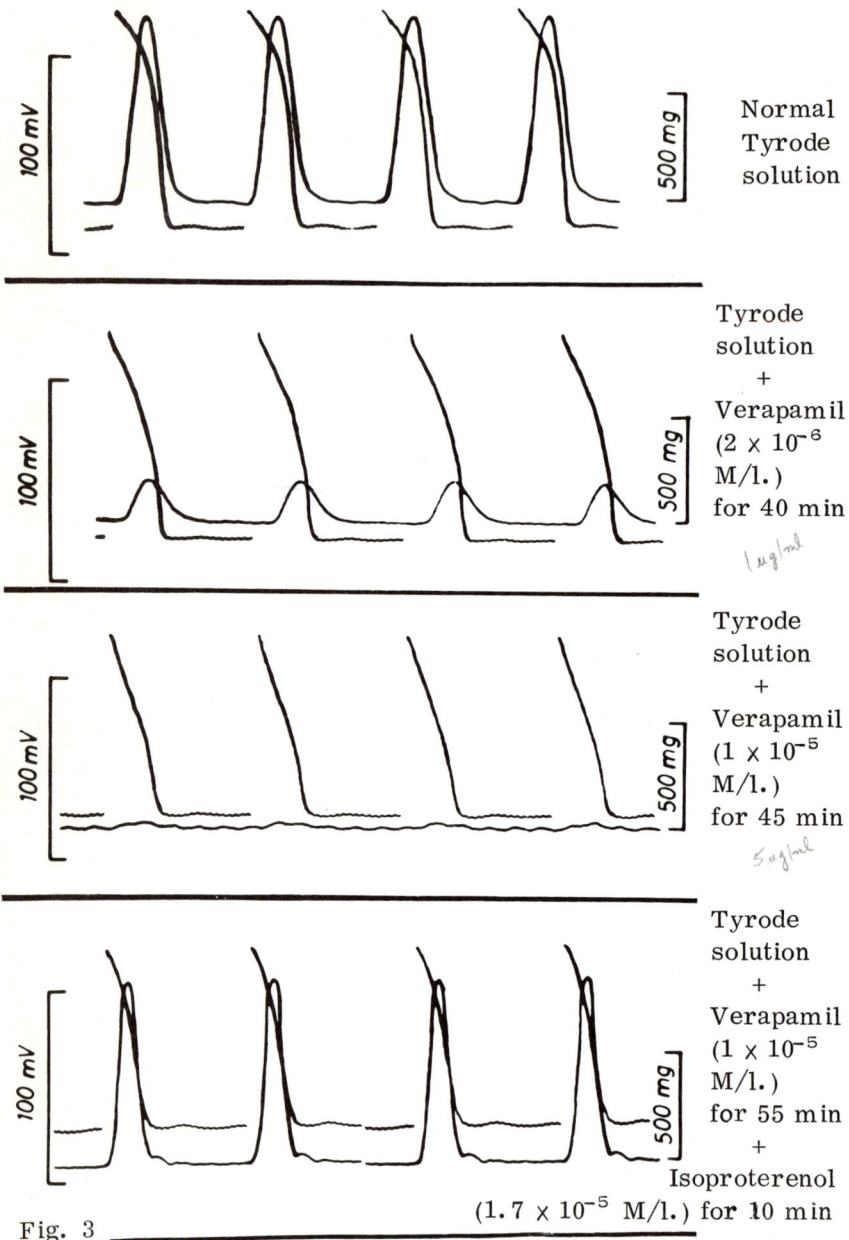

Fig. 3

Lindner[37] for prenylamine and by Haas et al.[22,23] for verapamil and compound D600. But the mechanism of action remained obscure until we found in 1964 that prenylamine and verapamil are capable of producing a similar selective loss of contractility as in Ca deficiency.[11] Later on it turned out that compound D600, a methoxy-derivative of verapamil, was several times more effective in antagonizing the Ca action than verapamil itself.[19] The most potent agent, however, is a new compound with the provisional name Bay a 1040: its chemical formula has not yet been officially disclosed. Fig. 3 shows, for example, that verapamil selectively abolishes, as all the specific Ca-antagonistic drugs do, the contractile response of a guinea-pig papillary muscle in a low concentration without any significant change in single fibre action potentials. In this experiment each molecule of verapamil antagonized approximately 200 Ca ions. This ratio in the case of compound D600 or compound Bay a 1040 is even higher: up to 1 to several thousand. The addition of calcium or, in the present experiment, isoproterenol restores the original height of the mechanical responses.

What is the mechanism of action of these powerful drugs? Tracer experiments, as well as measurements of the transmembrane Ca conductivity with the voltage-clamp technique, have demonstrated that verapamil, compound D600, and Bay a 1040

Fig. 3. Selective inhibition of cardiac contractility by verapamil, and the reversal of this effect by isoproterenol. Experiments on electrically-driven (2 shocks/sec) isolated papillary muscles of guinea-pigs. (From Fleckenstein.[12])

Transmembrane Ca inward current in normal Tyrode (2.2 mM Ca/l.)

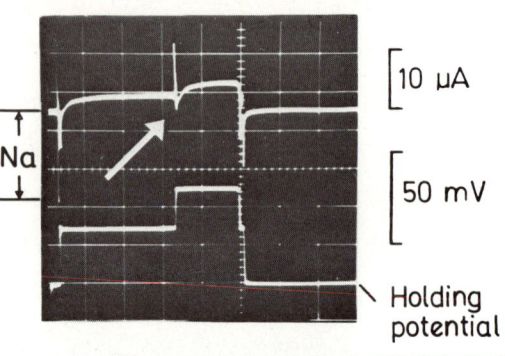

Complete disappearance of Ca inward current 10 min after addition of D600 (0.5 mg/l.)

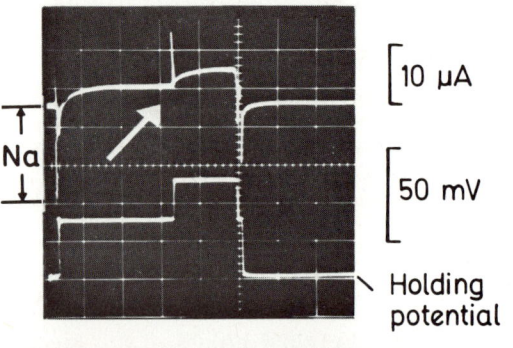

Overcompensation of the inhibitory effect of D600 on Ca inward current produced by addition of excess Ca (8.8 mM/l.)

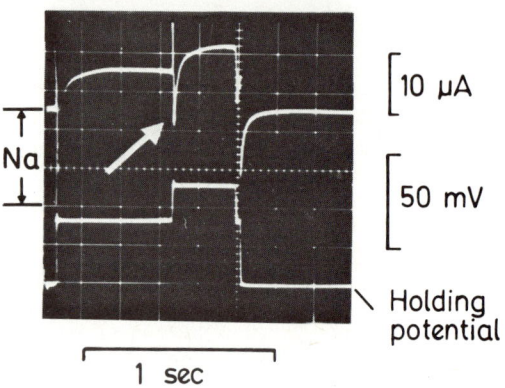

Fig. 4

block the transmembrane Ca influx into the excited heart muscle fibres but do not affect the simultaneous Na movements which are connected with the action potential (Fig. 4). Accordingly, under the influence of verapamil, compound D600 or Bay a 1040, the upstroke velocity and the height of the overshoot of the cardiac action potential, which indicate the transmembrane Na influx, remain practically constant in spite of the fact that the Ca-dependent contractile response has nearly disappeared (Fig. 5). Prenylamine proved to be somewhat less specific in its Ca antagonistic properties since it also reduces the Na inward current, and therefore the upstroke velocity of the cardiac action potential to some extent. Nevertheless, the interference of prenylamine with excitation-contraction coupling predominates.

It is evident from these results that the mammalian cardiac

Fig. 4. Measurements of the transmembrane Ca inward currents (downward deflections indicated by arrows) and of the rapid transient Na inward currents (marked on the left edge of the recordings) by the voltage-clamp technique. The experiments were carried out at 30° C on a right ventricular trabecula of a cat.

A. In a first step, the membrane potential was clamped for about 0.4 sec at a voltage which was 30 mV less negative than the original value. In this way the well known rapid transient Na inward current was elicited. Then, in a second step, the holding potential was further reduced by 20 mV. This causes the appearance of another inward current which is due to Ca influx.

B. D600 (0.5 mg/l.) blocks the Ca inward current completely without reducing the rapid transient Na current.

C. The effect of D600 is antagonized, and even overcompensated, by an increase in extracellular Ca up to 8.8 mM/l. (Unpublished observations of Kohlhardt, Physiological Institute, Freiburg, 1970.)

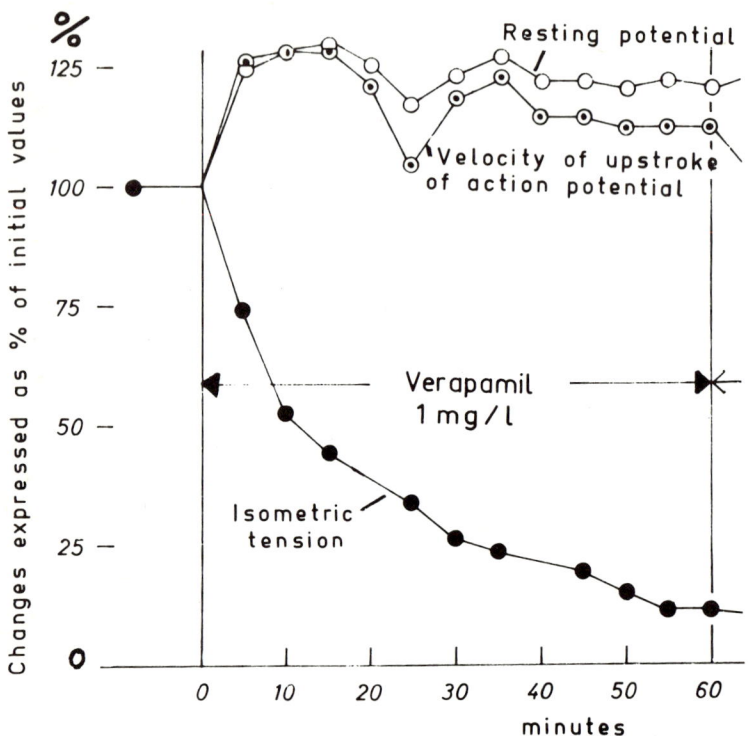

Fig. 5. Selective reduction of the Ca-dependent contractile force of a guinea-pig papillary muscle to one-tenth of normal by 1 mg/l. verapamil within 60 min, whilst the upstroke velocity and the height of the overshoot of the cardiac action potential, which indicate the transmembrane Na influx, did not decrease. Continuous microelectrode recordings were taken from the same cardiac fibre during 90 min. The absolute values (= 100%) at the beginning of the experiment were as follows: resting potential -75 mV; upstroke velocity 130 V/sec; isometric peak tension 700 mg; temp. 36° C; frequency of stimulation 2/sec. (Tritthart, Fleckenstein and Fleckenstein, 1968, unpublished.)

muscle fibre membranes have separate 'channels' for the Na- and for the Ca-influx. These channels can be blocked independently of each other. In this connection it is interesting to note that local anesthetics and other drugs with only Ca-antagonistic side-effects lack a distinct Ca specificity. Local anesthetics, for instance, do not discriminate between Ca and Na fluxes, or even interfere more with the Na movements than with the Ca transfer into the myocardium.

Since less ATP is consumed under the influence of Ca antagonistic inhibitors of excitation-contraction coupling, mechanical tension decreases while high-energy phosphates accumulate in the cardiac muscle. So the contractile failure produced by Ca-antagonistic drugs is always accompanied by an elevated creatine phosphate or ATP level and by a diminution in the orthophosphate fraction. This is true for the isolated myocardium as well as for hearts in situ after intravenous administration of Ca-antagonistic compounds. We have carried out several hundred experiments on guinea-pig hearts in situ (open chest preparations as in Figs. 6 and 7) in which the effects of large doses of a wide variety of specific and non-specific Ca-antagonistic drugs on heart diameter, contraction amplitude, cardiac frequency, and on arterial and venous blood pressure were investigated together with the changes in the high-energy phosphate content of the left ventricular myocardium. A summary of some of our biochemical results is given in Fig. 8. The graph shows that the creatine phosphate/inorganic phosphate ratio was consistently increased above normal when severe symptoms of heart incompetence appeared after intravenous administration

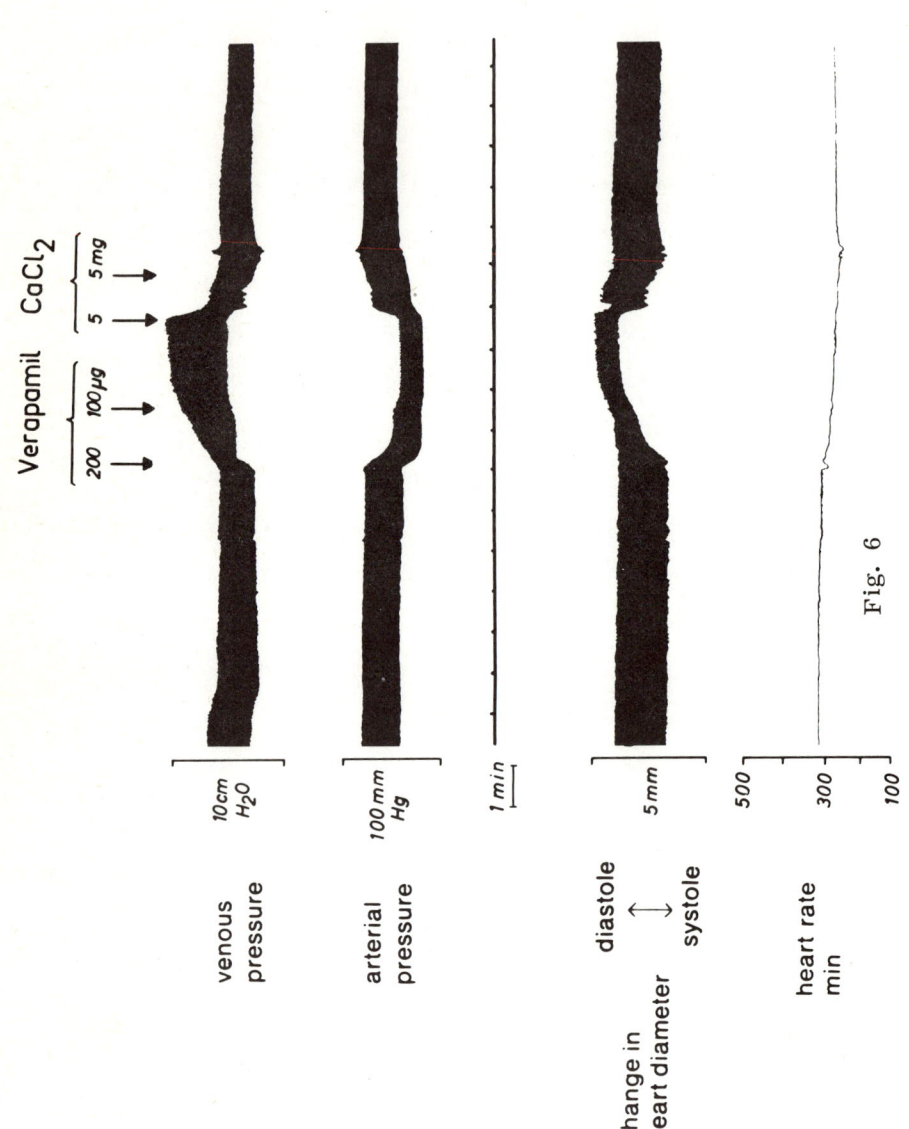

Fig. 6

of the Ca-antagonistic compounds. If, however, the high-energy phosphate consumption was restored by the administration of Ca (or by therapeutic doses of sympathomimetic amines or cardiac glycosides) the myocardial creatine phosphate/inorganic phosphate ratio rapidly fell to the normal range simultaneously with recovery of the contractile force.

Another consequence of the decrease in high-energy phosphate consumption is that the Ca-antagonistic drugs also reduce the cardiac oxygen requirement. The correlation between isometric tension and the additional consumption of oxygen due to mechanical activity is linear when, on rabbit papillary muscles, the extracellular Ca concentration is varied over the range 0-8 mM/l. (Fig. 9). Similarly, the Ca-antagonistic compounds are also capable of producing the same proportional change of isometric peak tension and extra consumption of oxygen if they are applied in different doses.[4] Fig. 10 shows, for instance, the proportional shift of

---

Fig. 6. Acute contractile failure of a guinea-pig heart (open chest preparation with the pericardium removed) after intravenous injection of a large overdose (1 mg/kg) of verapamil. Each increase in heart diameter (diastole, ventricular dilation) produces an upward deflection of the recording system,[32] whereas each downward movement means a decrease in heart diameter (systole, restoration of cardiac tonus). In many cases, acute ventricular dilation produced by specific or non-specific Ca-antagonistic compounds (see Fig. 8) was accompanied by a transient insufficiency of the tricuspid valve. Throughout the 700 open chest experiments of this standard type, suitable Statham elements were used for the blood pressure registration in the left jugular vein (P23 BB) and in the right carotid artery (P23 Db) under nembutal-ether anesthesia.[11, 15, 16]

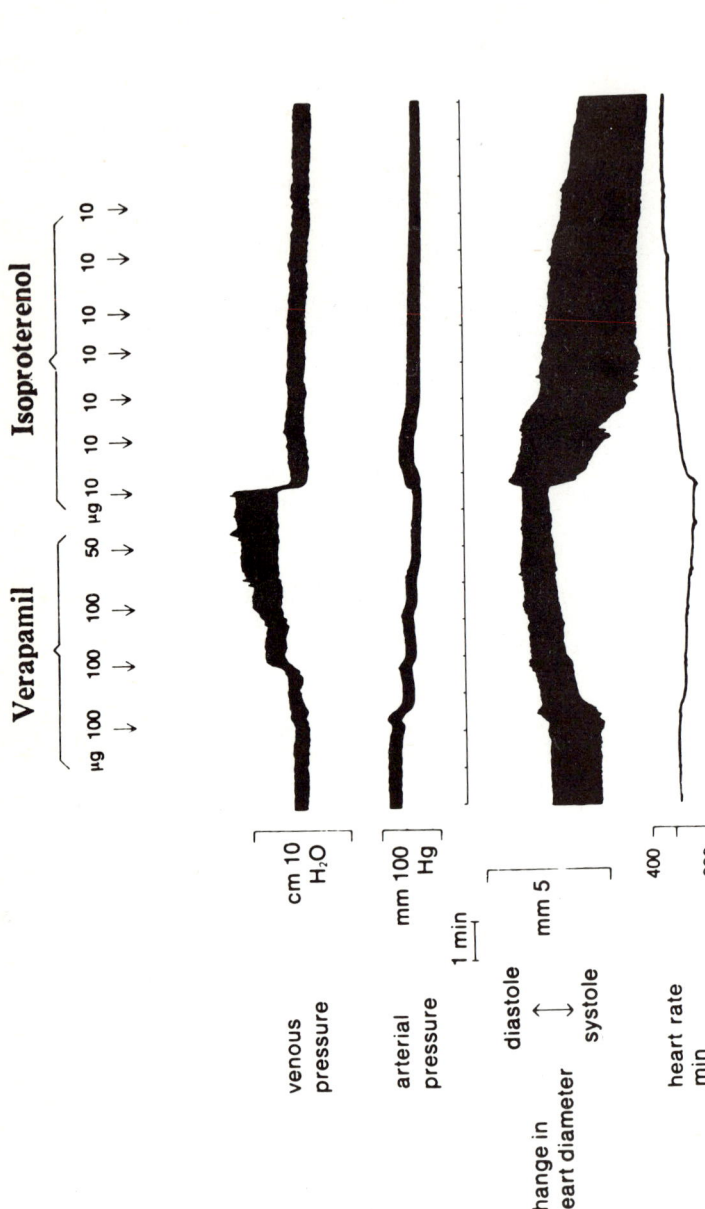

Fig. 7. Acute contractile failure of a guinea-pig heart produced by a large overdose (1.2 mg/kg) of verapamil (open chest preparation as in Fig. 6). After the first therapeutic dose of 10 μg isoproterenol (which corresponds to 35 μg/kg isoproterenol) contractility and venous blood pressure returned to normal within 20-30 sec. (From Fleckenstein.[11])

isometric tension and the additional consumption of oxygen under the influence of increasing concentrations of compound D600. Interestingly enough, a 50% reduction of contractile force and extra consumption of oxygen was produced, in this case, by a dose of D600 as low as 0.005 mg/l., i.e. a concentration of one part of the substance in 200 million parts of Tyrode solution. With a higher dose of D600 (1 mg/l.) both tension and oxygen consumption drop nearly to the resting level since the persisting electrical activity of the myocardial fibres influences the rate of respiration only to a rather insignificant extent. Nevertheless an appropriate dose of $CaCl_2$ will restore mechanical activity and oxygen consumption to normal even if previously the contractile system had been completely paralyzed.

The Ca-antagonistic inhibitors of excitation-contraction coupling are not only of academic interest since prenylamine and verapamil, for instance, are already widely used for therapeutic purposes in cases of angina pectoris and other forms of coronary disease. In such cases some restriction of the cardiac metabolism may be helpful in order to re-establish a suitable balance between a reduced coronary oxygen supply and the actual cardiac oxygen demand.

II. PROMOTERS OF EXCITATION-CONTRACTION COUPLING

Many observations have shown that the negative inotropic effects of Ca-antagonistic compounds can be neutralized not only by increasing the extracellular Ca concentration but also by the use of sympathomimetic amines or cardiac glycosides.[11, 15, 16, 18]

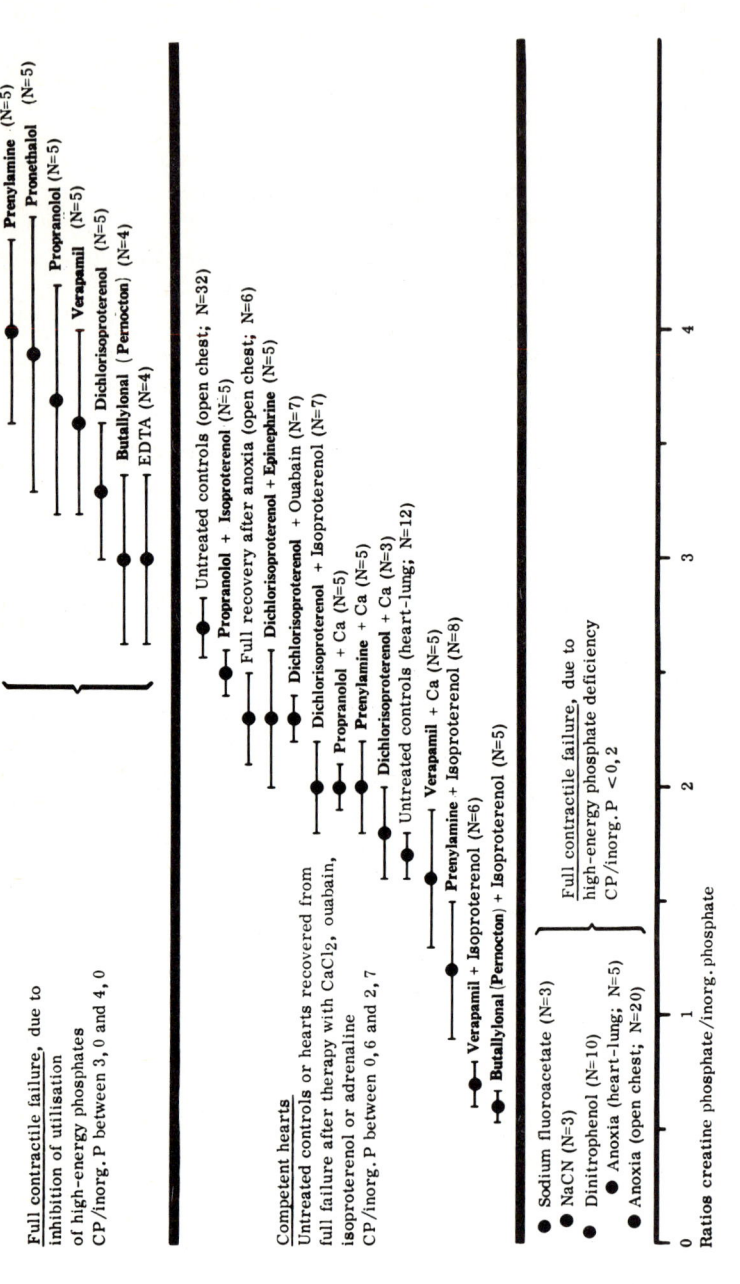

Fig. 8

Fig. 8. Increase of the creatine phosphate/inorganic phosphate ratio (up to a value of 3-4) in the left ventricular myocardium of guinea-pig hearts in situ during the contractile failure produced by inhibitors of excitation-contraction coupling. To cause this cardiac insufficiency the following large doses of specific Ca antagonists (6-12 mg/kg prenylamine; 0.4-1.0 mg/kg verapamil) or of several compounds with Ca antagonistic side effects (6-25 mg/kg dichloroisoproterenol; 3-5 mg/kg pronethalol; 1.5-6 mg/kg propranolol; 75 mg/kg butallylonal) or, as of EDTA (40-70 mg/kg) were administered intravenously in open chest experiments. If, however, the high-energy phosphate utilization was restored by $CaCl_2$ (45 mg/kg), isoproterenol (150 μg/kg), epinephrine (300 μg/kg) or ouabain (150-300 μg/kg), the creatine phosphate/inorganic phosphate ratio rapidly fell to the normal range pari passu with the recovery of the contractile tension. For comparison, the graph also shows the very low ratios (0.1-0.2) found in the left ventricular myocardium of rats under the influence of anoxia or metabolic poisons (10 mg/kg NaCN; 15 mg/kg sodium fluoroacetate; 30 mg/kg 2,4-dinitrophenol) when contractile failure developed due to a nearly complete high-energy phosphate exhaustion. The absolute concentrations of the acid-soluble phosphate compounds in 32 untreated control hearts in situ (expressed as μM/g blood free tissue wet weight) were as follows: creatine phosphate 8.3 (± 0.25),* inorganic phosphate 3.2 (± 0.11), ATP 4.6 (± 0.08), ADP 0.8 (± 0.03), total acid-soluble phosphorus 1160 (± 13) μg P/g. The corresponding control values for the left ventricular myocardium of 12 competent heart-lung preparations were: creatine phosphate 7.9 (± 0.2), inorganic phosphate 4.4 (± 0.05), ATP 4.6 (± 0.2), ADP 0.8 (± 0.03), total acid soluble phosphorus 1145 (± 21) μg P/g. (See Fleckenstein et al.[15])

---

*SE of mean.

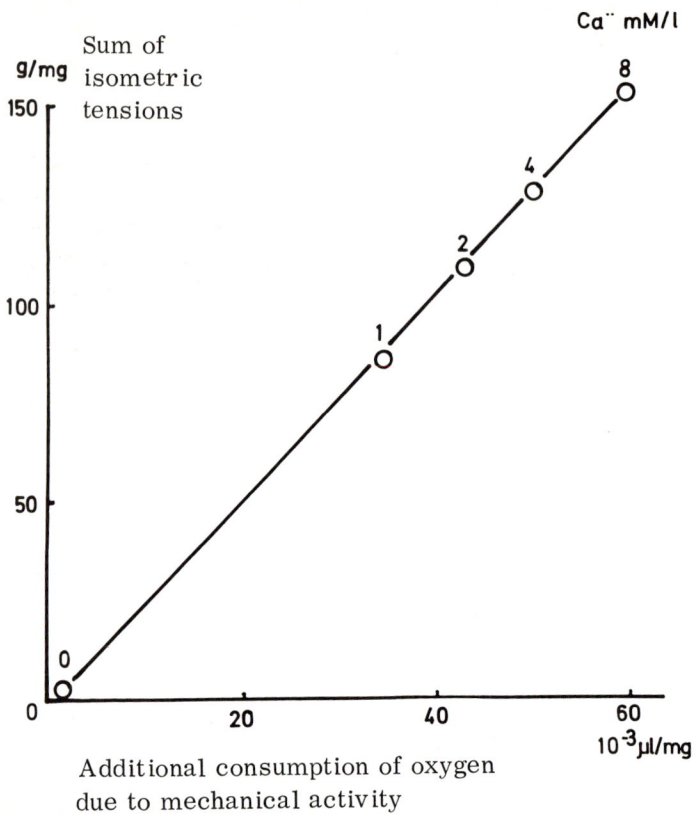

Fig. 9. Variation of extracellular Ca: Linear correlation between isometric tension and the additional consumption of oxygen due to mechanical activity (exceeding the oxygen uptake at rest) of a rabbit papillary muscle in Tyrode solutions of different Ca concentrations (0, 1, 2, 4 and 8 mM/l.). The muscle (1.6 mg wet weight) was incubated at rest in the different media each time for 20 min and then stimulated for 3.5 min at a frequency of 60/sec. Measurements of the rates of oxygen consumption (with a platinum electrode) and of mechanical tension (with a mechano-electronic displacement transducer) were made throughout the experiment at 30° C. The graph shows the sum of the isometric peak tensions produced during each stimulation period plotted against the corresponding additional consumptions of oxygen.[4]

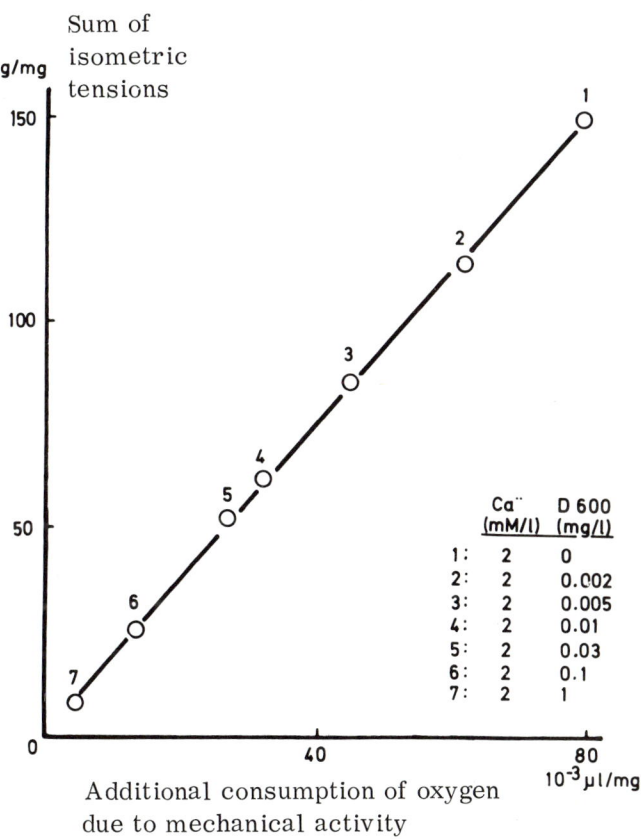

Fig. 10. Compound D600: Linear reduction of isometric tension and additional consumption of oxygen due to mechanical activity under the influence of increasing doses of the drug in Tyrode solution containing 2.0 mM Ca/l. (experimental procedure as in Fig. 9, rabbit papillary muscle, wet weight 1.1 mg, stimulation periods 3.0 minutes.[4]

Obviously these drugs influence the cardiac activity metabolism in the opposite direction to that of the Ca-antagonistic compounds since they intensify (or restore) the utilization of ATP for contraction, so that the mechanical tension as well as the oxygen requirement per heart beat will rise. However, even sympathomimetic catecholamines and cardiac glycosides seem to act, at least in part, through the mediation of Ca.

Otto Loewi[39] was the first to attribute the positive inotropic heart effects of digitalis glycosides to an interaction with Ca. But more than 40 years passed before Loewi's hypothesis was further substantiated.[20, 21, 27, 40, 50, 55] Recent experimental data suggest that cardiac glycosides facilitate the Ca release from sarcoplasmic or mitochondrial stores during excitation so that more free Ca is available to the contractile system.[35, 36] Similarly the positive inotropic action of sympathomimetic amines is caused by a potentiation of the Ca-dependent excitation-contraction coupling.[1] This effect is due to an increase of the Ca influx through the excited cardiac fibre membranes by sympathomimetic amines such as epinephrine[42] or isoproterenol, according to our results (see Section III). Among the sympathomimetic amines tested isoproterenol was by far the most potent Ca promoter. In all cases of contractile failure produced by a simple Ca withdrawal or by Ca antagonistic inhibitors of excitation-contraction coupling, isoproterenol was capable of restoring high-energy phosphate utilization and contractile tension with a minimum Ca requirement (see Figs. 3, 7 and 8). It is interesting to note that caffeine can also reverse the metabolic and mechanical effects of Ca-antagonistic compounds.[15]

III. INTRACELLULAR Ca OVERLOAD LEADING TO HIGH-ENERGY PHOSPHATE DEFICIENCY AS AN ETIOLOGICAL FACTOR IN THE PRODUCTION OF MYOCARDIAL FIBRE NECROSES

The catecholamine-induced increase of Ca influx and of cardiac high-energy phosphate consumption has also some important pathological consequences. We were able to show two years ago on rats that large doses of sympathetic amines, particularly isoproterenol, not only cause an excessive Ca uptake but also initiate a dangerous fall in the high-energy phosphate content of heart muscle.[13, 17] Fig. 11 shows the changes in the ATP, creatine phosphate and orthophosphate content of the left ventricular myocardium of 90 rats during an observation period of 24 hours following a single subcutaneous injection of 30 mg/kg isoproterenol. This dose produces a 50% loss of ATP and an 85% loss of creatine phosphate within two hours. And later on, in all cases, the high-energy phosphate exhaustion was followed by the development of disseminated or confluent myocardial fibre necroses. Such isoproterenol-induced cardiac lesions were first described by Rona et al.[43] but the etiology remained obscure. As pointed out by Stanton and Schwartz,[53] the following hypotheses have been proposed.

1) Cardiac hypoxemia may result from isoproterenol-induced hypotension accompanied by increased cardiac work and enhanced myocardial oxygen demands.[43]
2) Dilation of precapillary shunts may cause blood to bypass the capillary circulation and induce endocardial ischemia.[24]

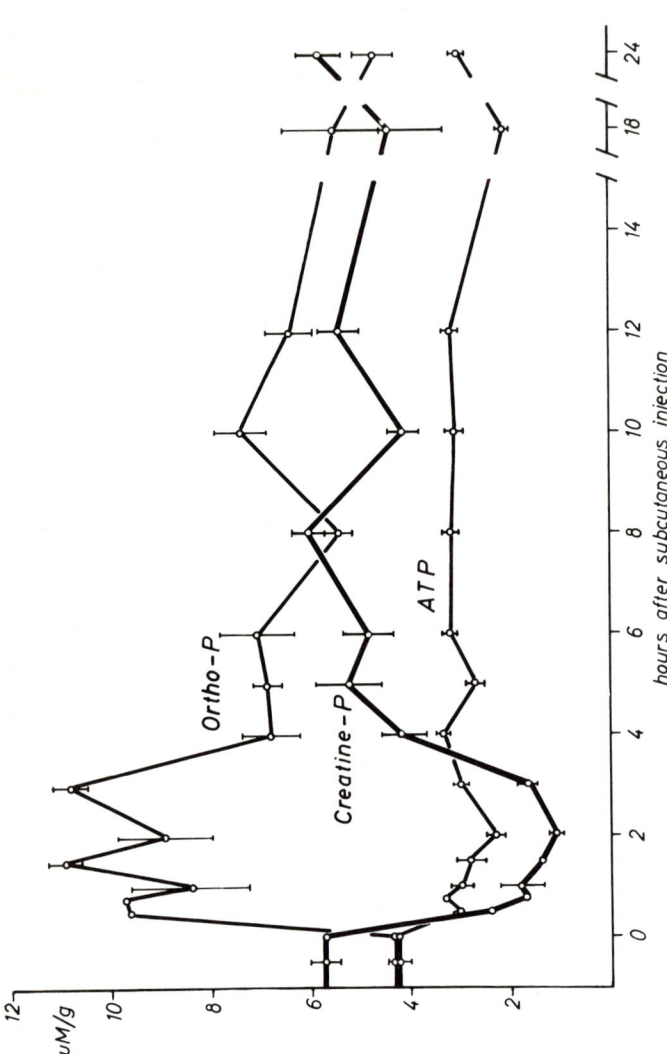

Fig. 11. Isoproterenol-induced changes in the concentrations of ATP, creatine phosphate and orthophosphate in the left ventricular myocardium of 90 rat hearts after subcutaneous injection of 30 mg/kg isoproterenol during an observation period of 24 hr. (From Fleckenstein et al.[17])

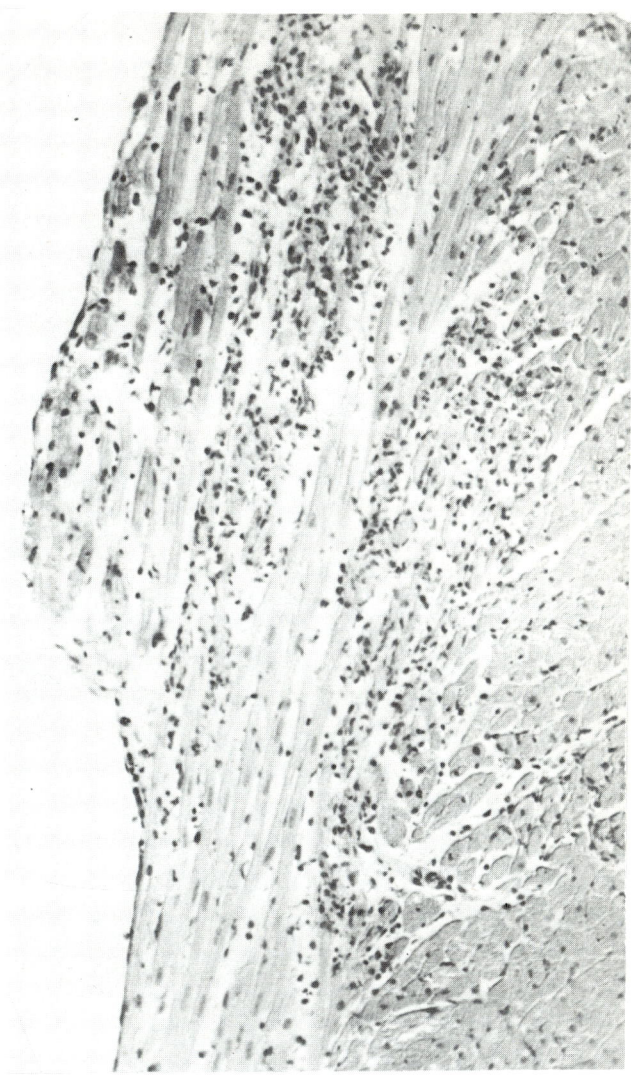

Fig. 12A: Myocardial necroses in the right ventricular wall of a rat 24 hr after subcutaneous administration of isoproterenol (30 mg/kg).

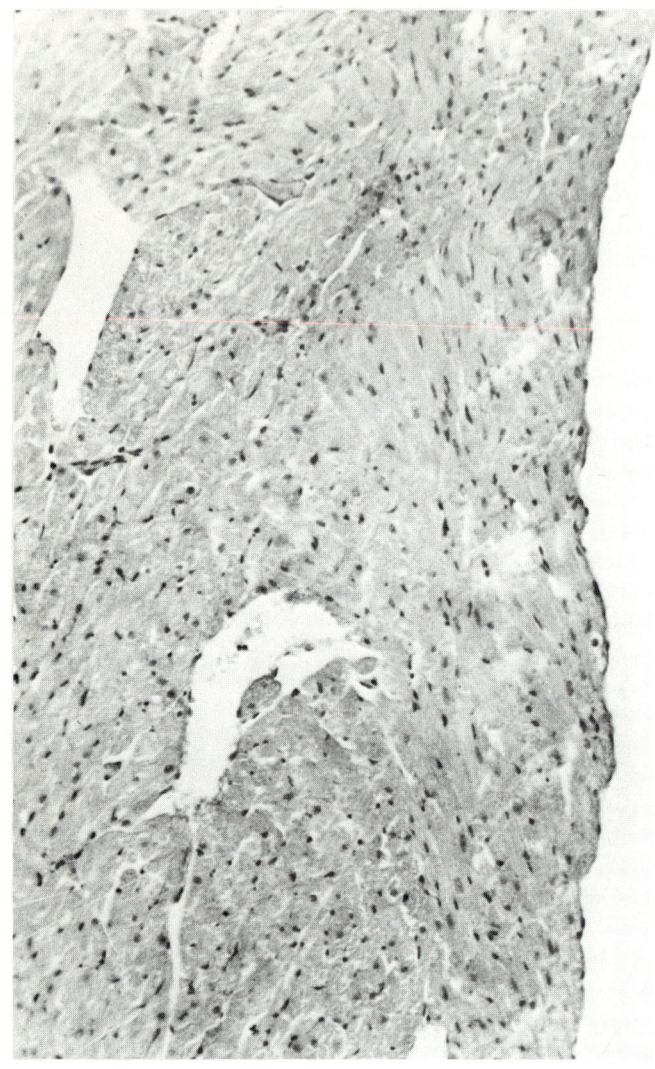

Fig. 12B: Protection from the isoproterenol effect shown in A by the simultaneous s.c. injection of 50 mg/kg verapamil. Hematoxylin-eosin stain. [13]

3) Hypoxia may result from direct, metabolic, oxygen-wasting actions of catecholamines on the heart.[41]

4) Hyperlipidemia may elicit, in an unidentified manner, alterations in cell membrane permeability which induce myocardial lesions.[46]

5) Cardiac necrosis may occur because of local potassium loss from the cardiac cell.[47]

However, none of these hypotheses can explain the fact that Ca-antagonistic compounds such as verapamil, D600, or prenylamine are capable of protecting the rat heart against structural damage if given in appropriate dosage at the same time as the isoproterenol (see Figs. 12-14 from Fleckenstein[13,17]). Therefore, one has to assume that the crucial point in the production of myocardial lesions consists of an isoproterenol-induced Ca overload of the myocardial fibres leading to a pronounced high-energy phosphate deficiency which can be prevented by Ca-antagonistic drugs. It is obvious that the maintenance and permanent restitution of the cells depend on the availability of sufficient amounts of ATP and CP for many energy-consuming synthetic processes which are involved in regeneration of the living structure. But isoproterenol, by producing a severe and long-lasting high-energy phosphate exhaustion, interferes with these vital reactions so that the survival of the cardiac tissue becomes difficult and, for many fibres, even impossible. In this respect the energetic situation of the myocardium of isoproterenol-treated animals closely resembles the metabolic state of the heart muscle in anoxia, ischemia, or under the influence of metabolic poisons, such as cyanide or

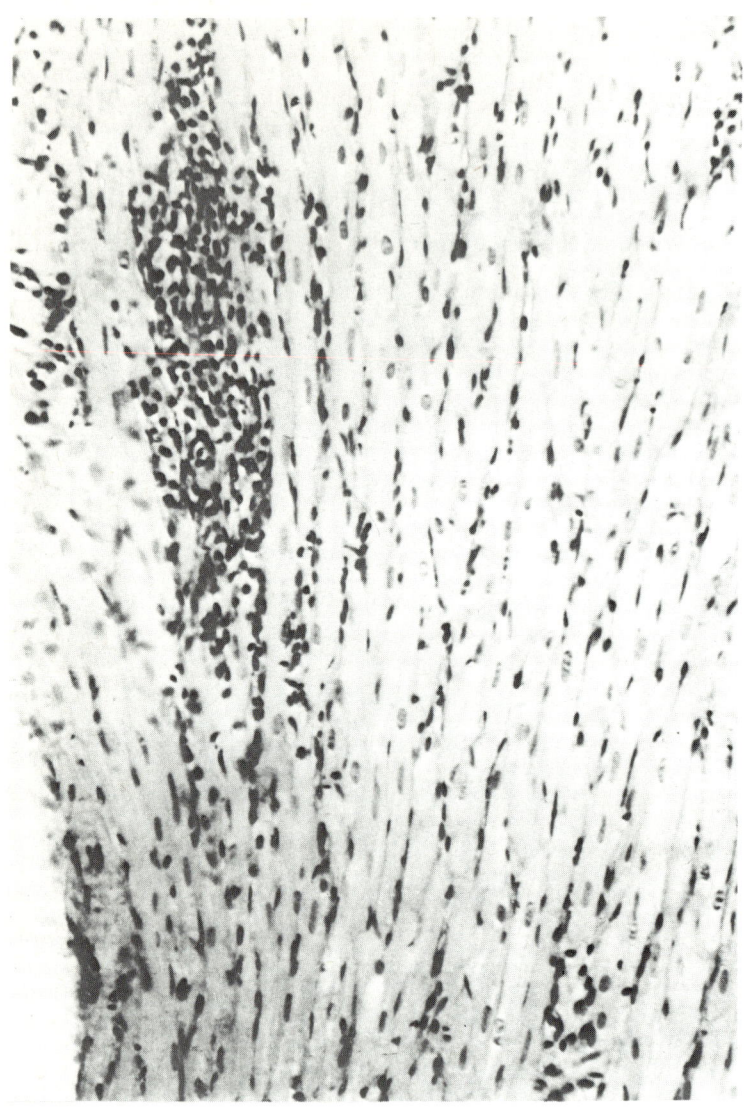

Fig. 13A: Myocardial fibre necroses in the left ventricular wall of a rat 24 hr after subcutaneous administration of isoproterenol (30 mg/kg).

Fig. 13B: Protection from the isoproterenol effect shown in A by the simultaneous subcutaneous injection of 100 mg/kg prenylamine. Hematoxylin-eosin stain. (Leder and Fleckenstein, unpublished.)

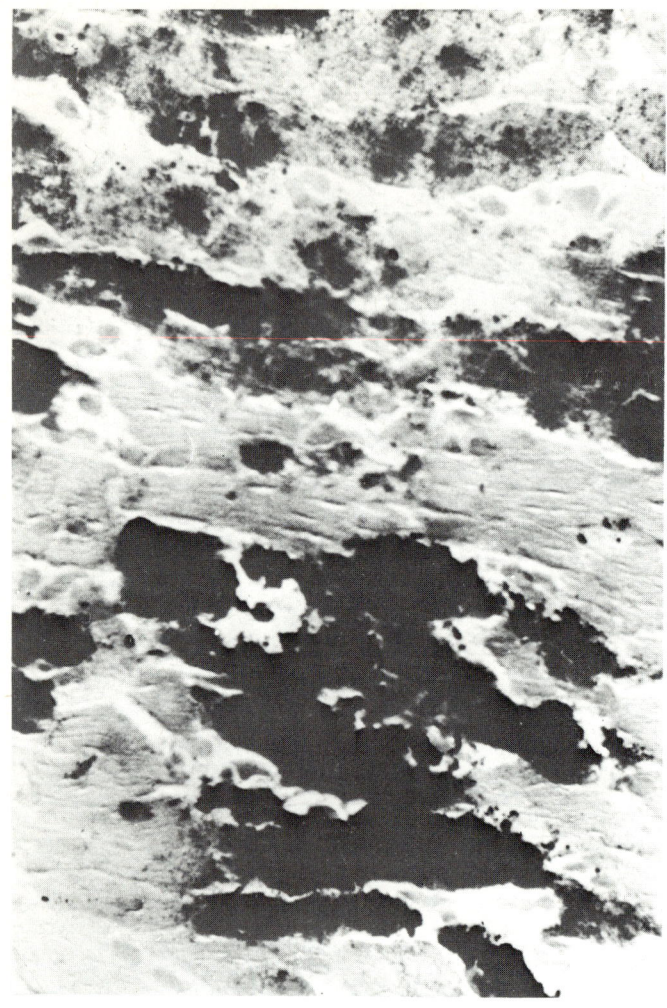

Fig. 14A: Occurrence of Ca deposits, represented by the black areas, in the right ventricular wall of a rat 3 hr after the subcutaneous injection of 30 mg/kg isoproterenol.

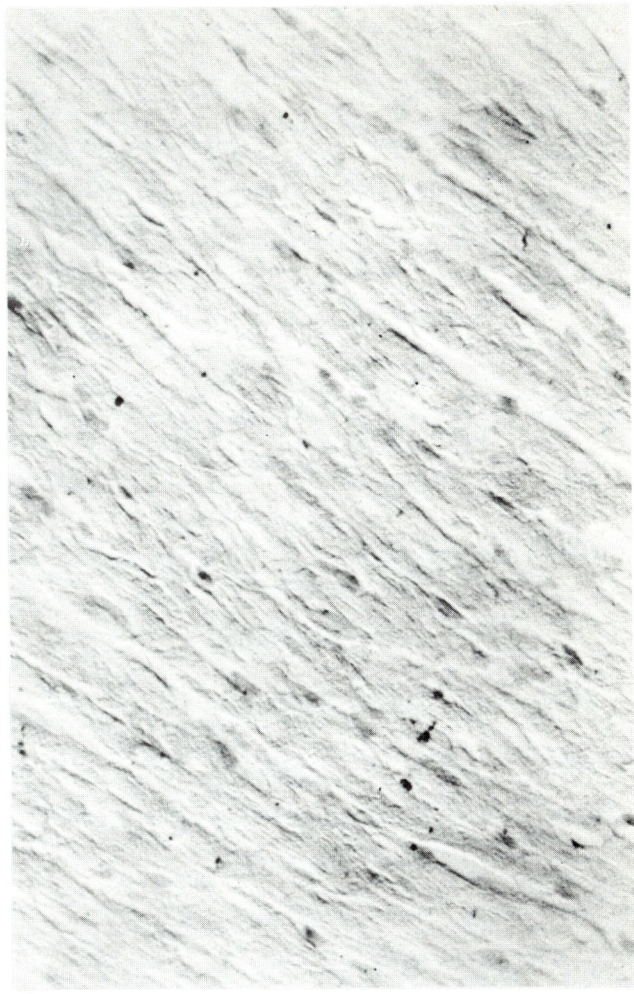

Fig. 14B: Protection from the isoproterenol effect shown in A by the simultaneous subcutaneous administration of 20 mg/kg D600. (v. Kossa's stain for Ca salts.)[13]

2, 4-dinitrophenol, since in all these cases cardiac function and structural integrity cannot be maintained if the creatine phosphate pool is nearly empty. Moreover, with less than 40% of the normal ATP content, no survival or reanimation of a heart is possible according to observations in our laboratory.[31] So the loss of ATP seems to be as critical as the creatine phosphate breakdown. Ca-antagonistic compounds, on the other hand, protect the hearts against the deleterious effects of an overdose of catecholamines by stabilizing the ATP and creatine phosphate concentrations at a sufficiently high level. As shown in Fig. 15, compound D600 (20 mg/kg) or verapamil (50 mg/kg) are fully effective in inhibiting the isoproterenol-induced breakdown of the creatine phosphate fraction in the left ventricular myocardium of rats. Similar effects were obtained with a single subcutaneous dose (250 mg/kg) of prenylamine. Due to slow absorption of prenylamine, this route of administration was probably not very suitable, but nevertheless the protective action of prenylamine against high-energy phosphate exhaustion and myocardial lesions proved to be satisfactory.

Further evidence for a close interrelationship between myocardial Ca overload, high-energy phosphate deficiency, and the production of cardiac necroses was obtained in experiments on rats with Ca^{45}. All animals received an intraperitoneal injection of 1 μC Ca^{45}/100 g body weight.* As shown in Fig. 16, the radioactivity of the left and right ventricular myocardium keeps at a

---

*Preliminary reports about our results with radiocalcium were given in previous papers.[14, 28-30]

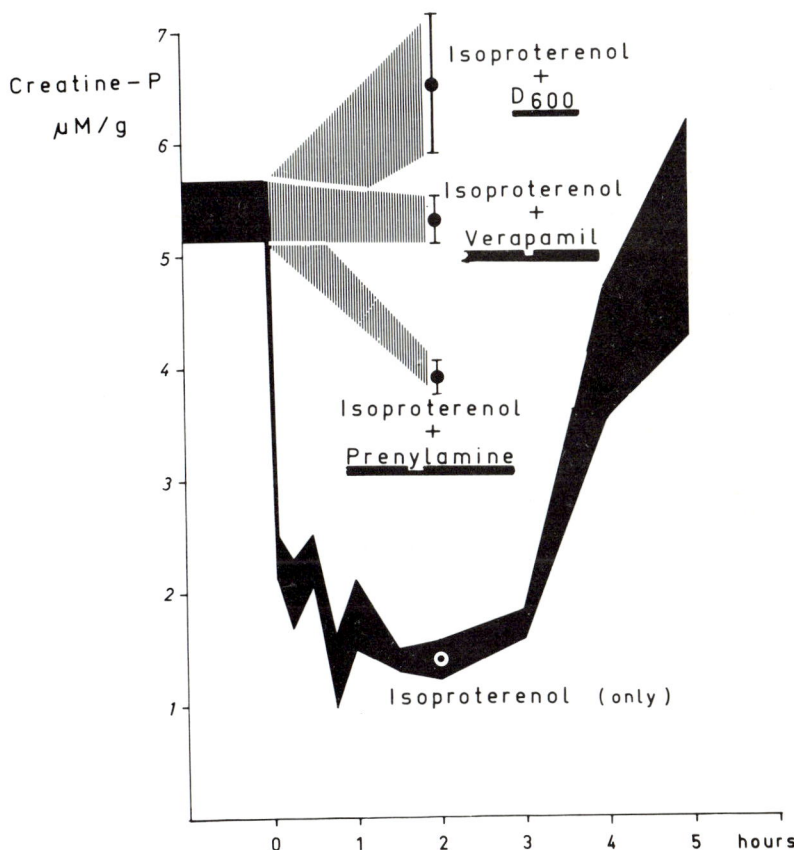

Fig. 15. Inhibition of the isoproterenol-induced creatine phosphate breakdown in the left ventricular myocardium of rats by three Ca antagonistic compounds. The drugs were applied simultaneously by single subcutaneous injections at separate sites. The following doses were administered: isoproterenol (30 mg/kg), verapamil (50 mg/kg), compound D600 (20 mg/kg), prenylamine (250 mg/kg).[17]

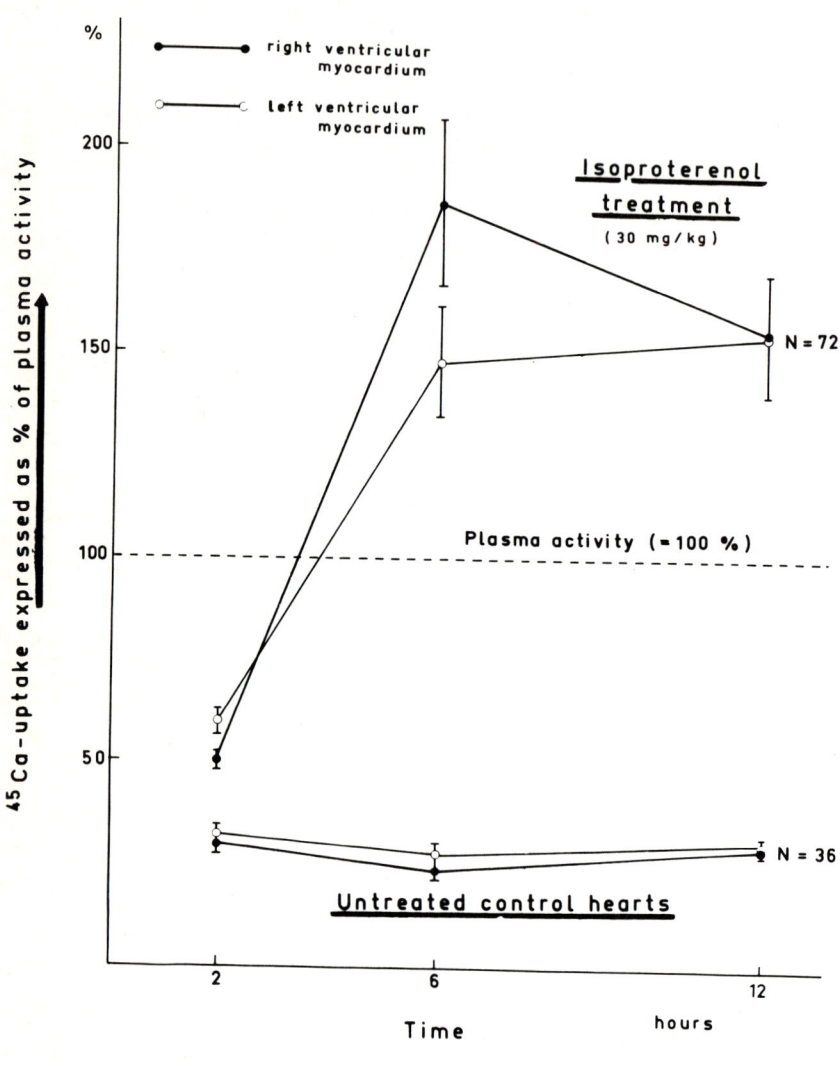

Fig. 16

constant value (about 25% of the radiocalcium activity of the plasma) during an observation period of 12 hours. But after subcutaneous administration of 30 mg/kg isoproterenol, the net Ca^{45} uptake into the myocardial fibres is increased by a factor of 6 to 10 with a maximum at six hours. Such hearts developed severe disseminated necroses. The Ca-antagonistic inhibitors of excitation-contraction coupling, on the other hand, can block the excessive isoproterenol-induced Ca^{45} incorporation into the right and left ventricular myocardium if the drugs are simultaneously administered with the isoproterenol. The doses of verapamil, D600 or prenylamine which inhibit an excessive Ca^{45} uptake are identical with those preventing high-energy phosphate exhaustion and myocardial lesions (see Figs. 17 and 18).

Another type of experiment is shown in Fig. 19. The graphs represent log dose-response curves of the isoproterenol-induced radiocalcium uptake into the right ventricular myocardium of rats. The measurements were made six hours after subcutaneous injections of different doses of the drug. The rise in Ca^{45} uptake above the control level begins with an isoproterenol dose as small as 0.1 mg/kg and proceeds steeply to a maximum which is beyond the high dose of 30 mg/kg. Again the Ca antagonistic compounds

Fig. 16. Increase of the net radiocalcium uptake into the left and right ventricular myocardium of rats produced by the subcutaneous injection of 30 mg/kg isoproterenol. The Ca^{45} uptake into 1 g of fresh cardiac tissue is expressed as a percentage of the corresponding Ca^{45} activity in 1 ml of plasma during an observation period of 12 hr after intraperitoneal administration of 1 µC Ca^{45} per 100 g body weight.

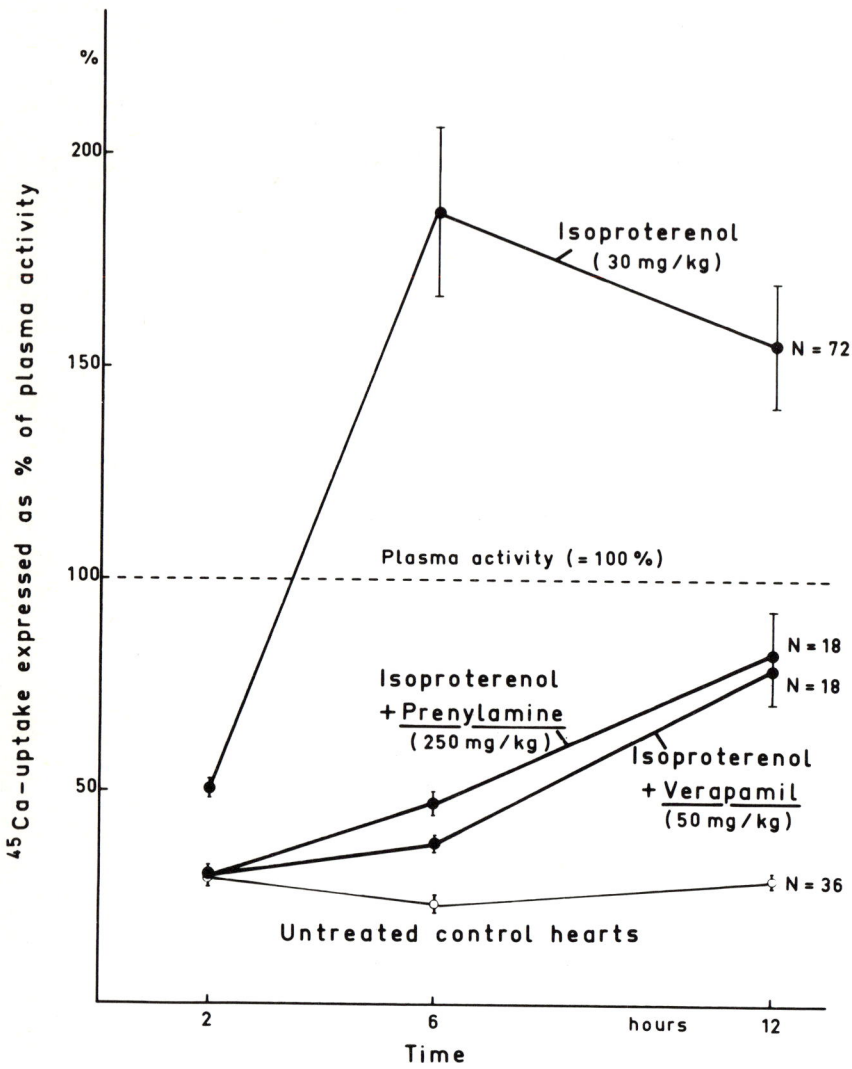

Fig. 17. Inhibition of the isoproterenol-induced net Ca^{45} uptake by 50 mg/kg verapamil or 250 mg/kg prenylamine in the right ventricular myocardium of rats (method as in Fig. 16).

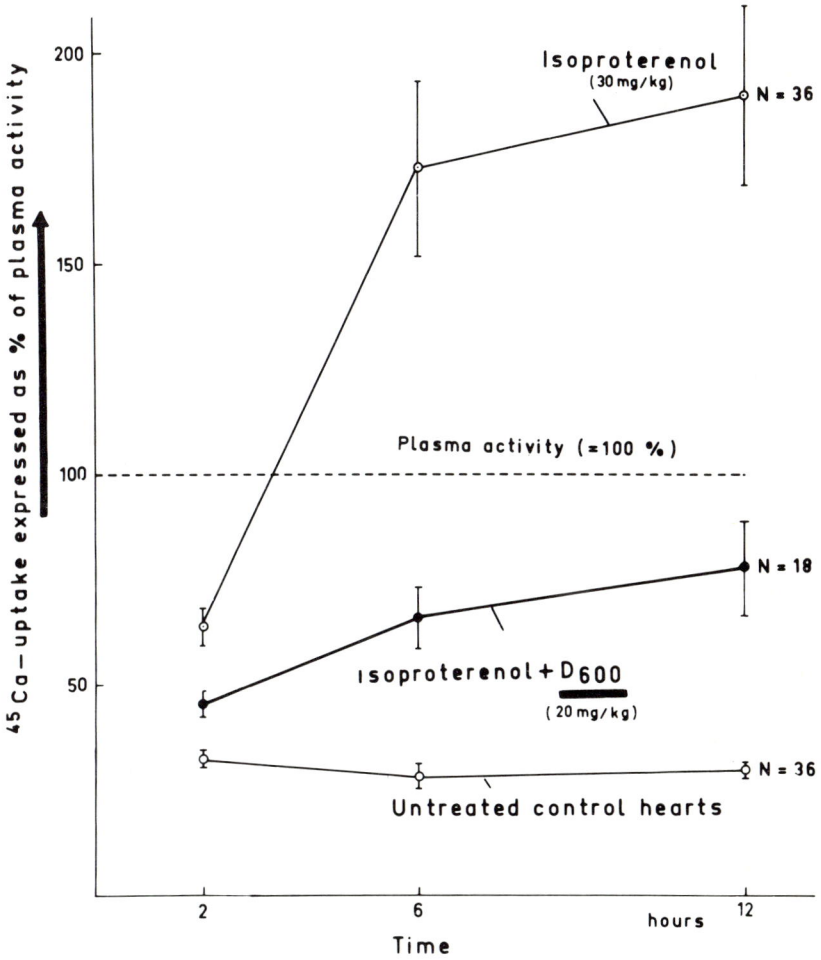

Fig. 18. Inhibition of the isoproterenol-induced net Ca^{45} uptake by 20 mg/kg D600 in the left ventricular myocardium (apical region) of rats (method as in Fig. 16).

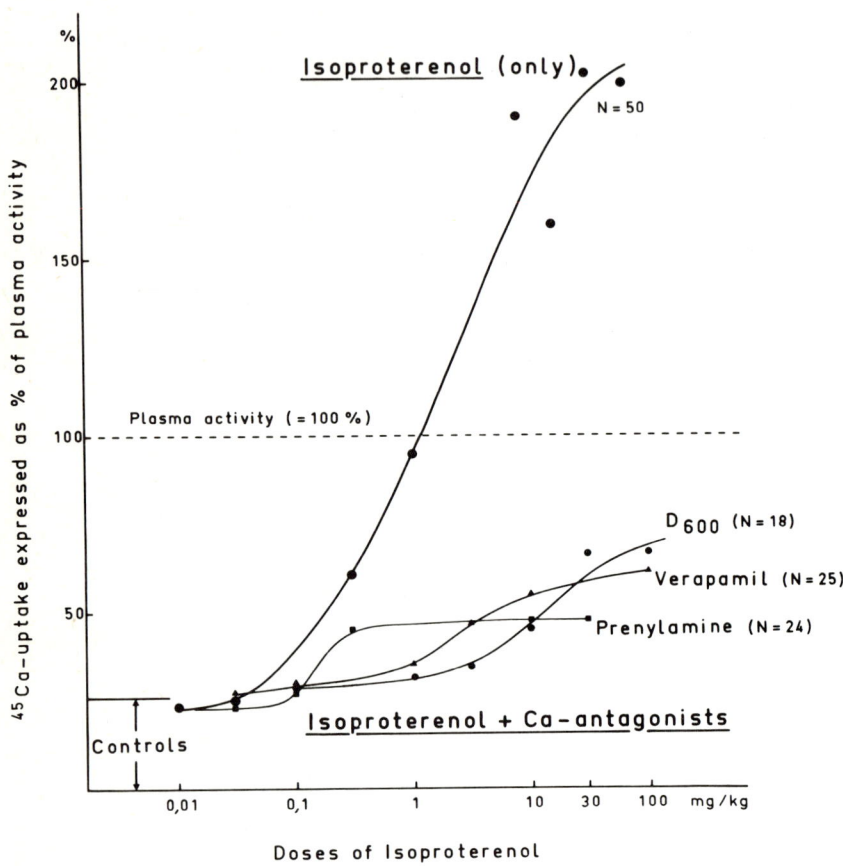

Fig. 19. Log dose-response curves of the isoproterenol-induced radiocalcium uptake into the right ventricular myocardium of rats obtained with or without simultaneous administration of three Ca antagonistic compounds (10 mg/kg D600, 17 mg/kg verapamil, 250 mg/kg prenylamine). All measurements were made 6 hr after subcutaneous injection of the drugs.

verapamil (17 mg/kg), D600 (10 mg/kg) or prenylamine (250 mg/kg) neutralize the isoproterenol effects to a rather impressive extent. Small doses of isoproterenol are completely blocked whilst higher doses (up to 100 mg/kg) are greatly reduced in their action.

In this connection it is highly interesting to note that KCl or $MgCl_2$, given orally, is also capable of inhibiting the excessive isoproterenol-induced radiocalcium incorporation into the myocardial fibres. Obviously K and Mg ions are physiological Ca antagonists which can also protect the heart against the deleterious Ca overload. Figs. 20 and 21 show experimental data obtained on the left ventricular myocardium of rats. It is evident from these observations that even one single oral dose of KCl or $MgCl_2$ can enormously depress the dose-response curve of the isoproterenol-induced Ca^{45} uptake. Our results explain the important findings of Selye,[51] Bajusz[3] and others who have studied, years ago, the beneficial influence of K and Mg salts in preventing experimental cardiac fibre necroses of different types. The production of isoproterenol-induced cardiac lesions was also shown to be inhibited by KCl.[40] Our own histological observations are in good harmony with this earlier work.

In their investigations about the factors which prevent or enhance myocardial necrotization, Selye and Bajusz have also discovered that rats can be sensitized for the production of cardiac necroses by pretreatment with certain corticosteroids, dihydrotachysterol or NaH_2PO_4. The same substances aggravate the cardiotoxicity of isoproterenol.[44] Therefore we have also examined how these sensitizing substances influence the radiocalcium uptake.

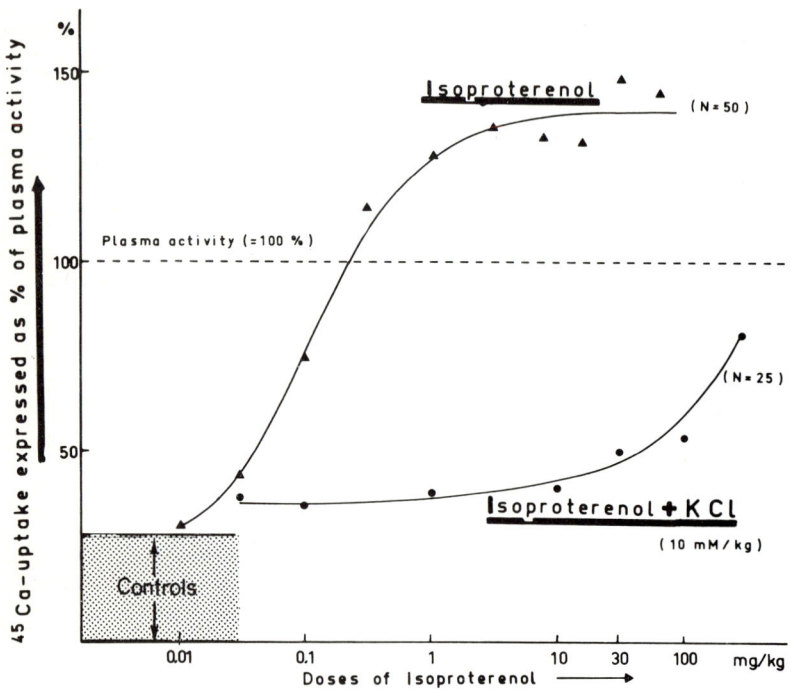

Fig. 20. Prevention of the excessive isoproterenol-induced Ca^{45} uptake into the inner layer of the left ventricular myocardium of rats by a single oral standard dose of KCl (10 mM/kg). The log dose-response curves were obtained 6 hr after subcutaneous injection of different amounts of isoproterenol with or without KCl.

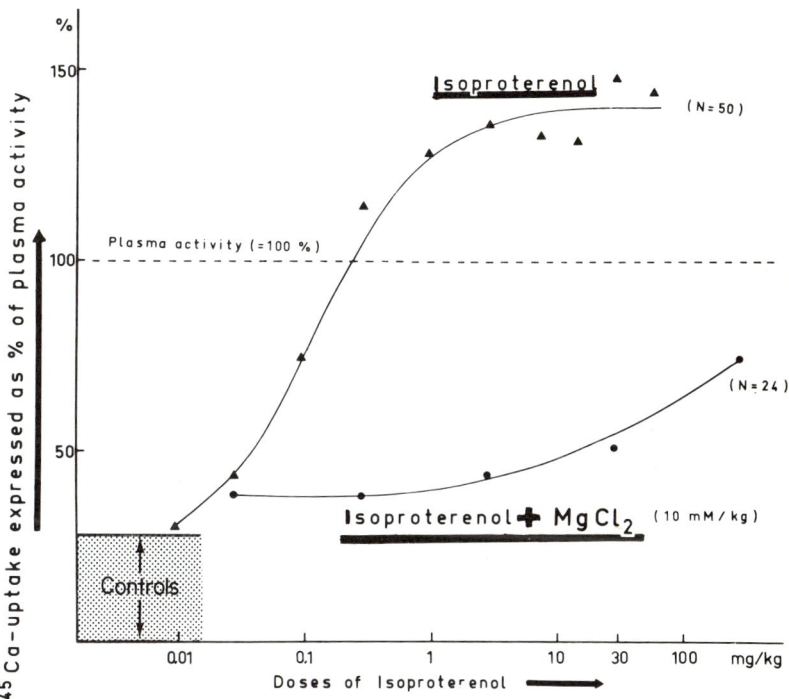

Fig. 21. Prevention of the excessive isoproterenol-induced Ca^{45} uptake into the inner layer of the left ventricular myocardium of rats by a single oral standard dose of $MgCl_2$ (10 mM/kg). The log dose-response curves were obtained 6 hr after subcutaneous injection of different amounts of isoproterenol with or without $MgCl_2$.

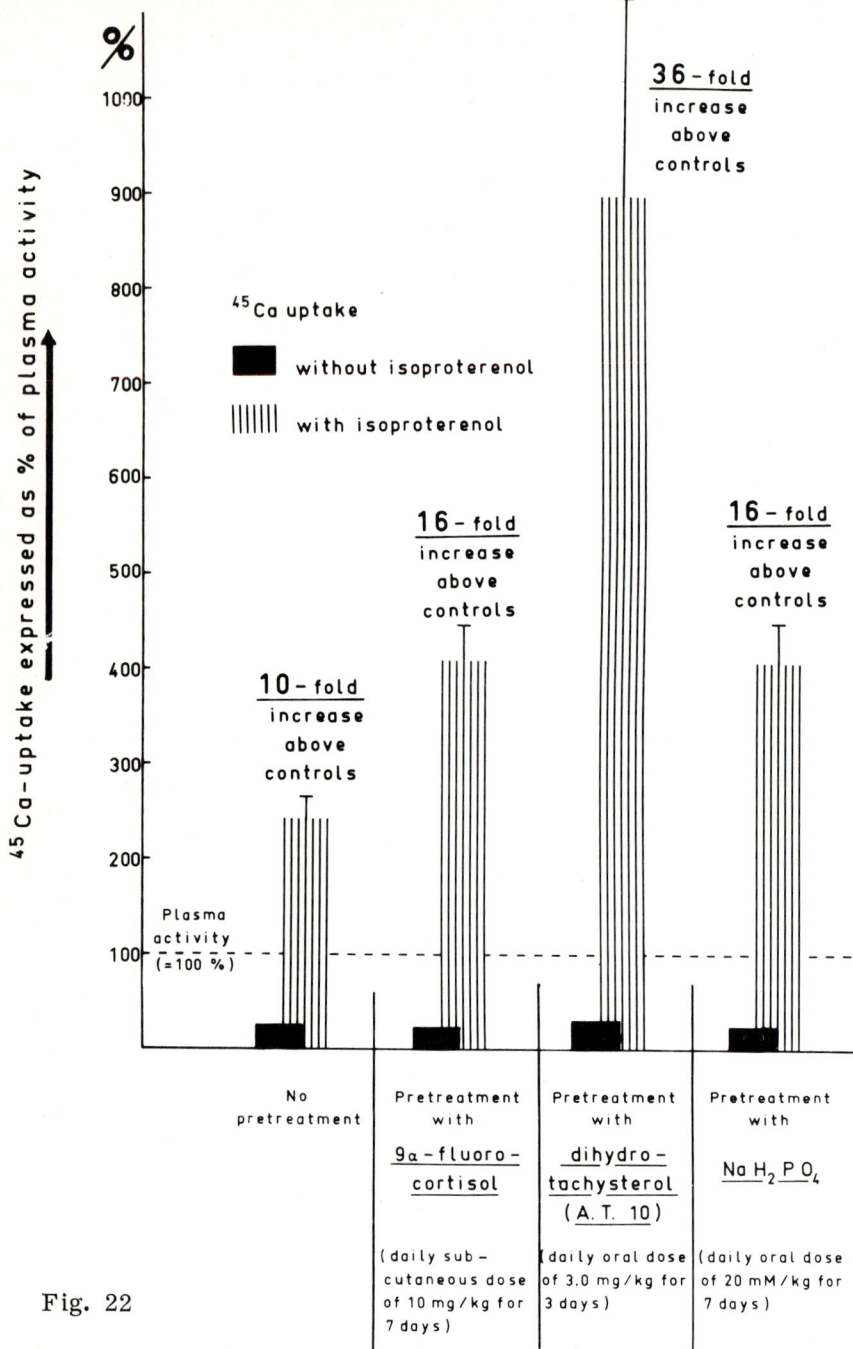

Fig. 22

Fig. 22 shows that 9α-fluorocortisol acetate, dihydrotachysterol (AT 10), or monosodium phosphate have apparently no effect of their own on the cardiac radiocalcium incorporation. But if isoproterenol is administered after pretreatment with these sensitizing agents, a tremendous increase in the radiocalcium uptake occurs. The maximum was reached in the hearts of dihydrotachysterol-pretreated rats six hours after administration of 30 mg/kg isoproterenol, when the radiocalcium accumulation was found to be 36 times greater than the normal control value. After sensitization by 9-α-fluorocortisol acetate or NaH_2PO_4, the increase was 16-fold. The structural damage in these hearts was extremely severe. But, even in this situation, the radiocalcium uptake as well as the number and size of the necroses can be greatly diminished with the help of Ca-antagonistic drugs or by oral administration of KCl or $MgCl_2$.[24] Our results demonstrate that the aggravation of the cardiotoxic response to isoproterenol in animals pretreated with 9-α-fluorocortisol acetate, dihydrotachysterol, or NaH_2PO_4 is closely correlated with a potentiation of the isoproterenol-induced Ca accumulation. This excessive Ca overload produces a massive deficiency of the cardiac high-energy phosphates. As shown in Figs. 23 and 24, pretreatment with 9-α-fluorocortisol acetate, for instance, leads to further accentuation and prolongation of the

---

Fig. 22. Sensitization to the isoproterenol-induced radiocalcium uptake into the right ventricular myocardium of rats by pretreatment with 9α-fluorocortisol acetate, dihydrotachysterol or NaH_2PO_4. All measurements were carried out 6 hr after subcutaneous administration of isoproterenol (30 mg/kg).

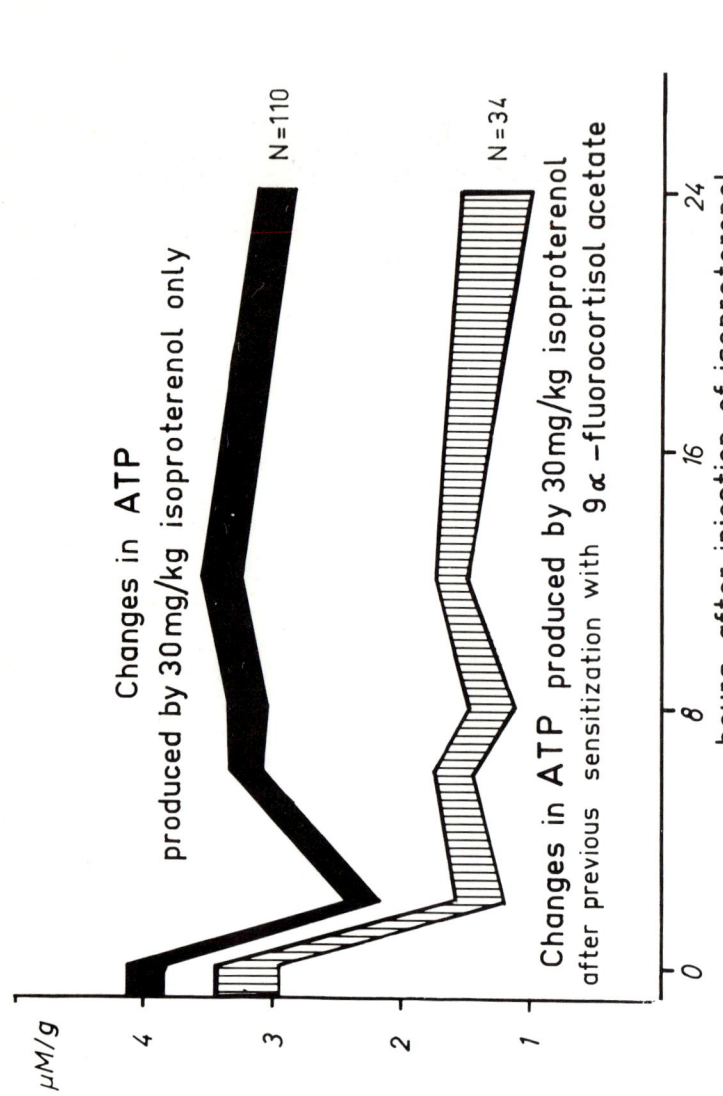

Fig. 23. Accentuation of the isoproterenol-induced fall in the ATP content of the left ventricular myocardium of rats by pretreatment with 9α-fluorocortisol acetate. For the sensitization of the animals a daily dose of 10 mg/kg 9α-fluorocortisol acetate was administered subcutaneously for successive 7 days. (Döring and Fleckenstein, unpublished.)

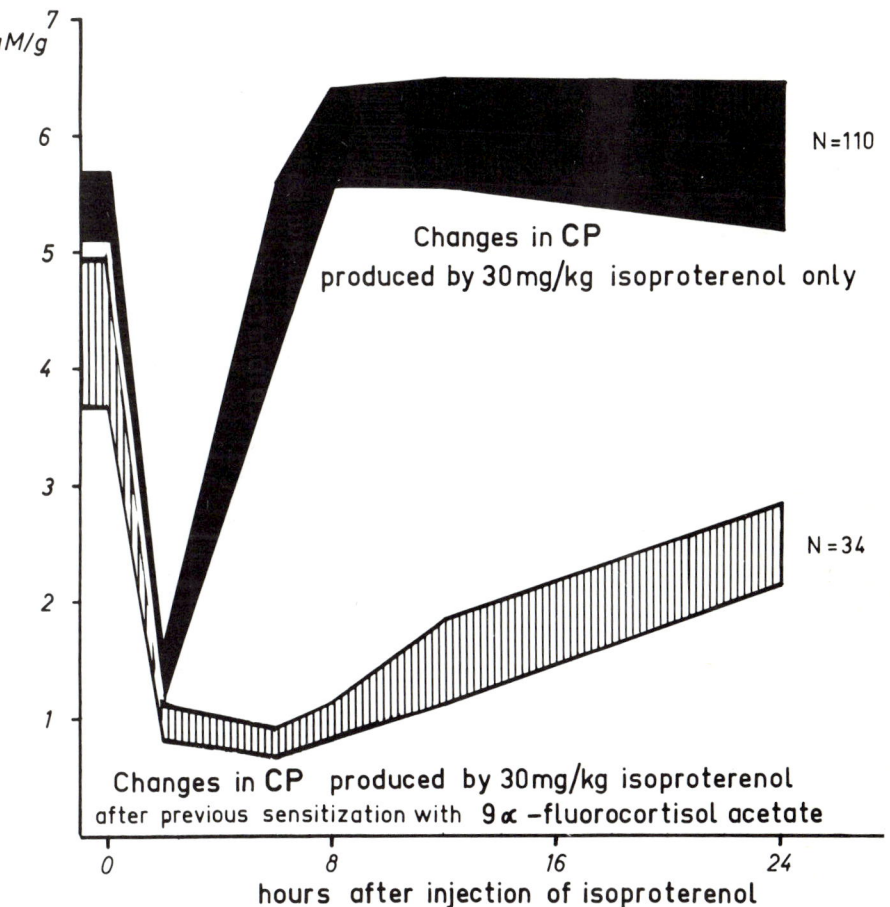

Fig. 24. Accentuation and prolongation of the isoproterenol-induced creatine phosphate (CP) deficiency by pretreatment with 9α-fluorocortisol acetate. The determinations of the CP content were carried out on the same specimens of cardiac tissue as the ATP analysis in Fig. 23. (Döring and Fleckenstein, unpublished.)

isoproterenol-induced fall in the myocardial ATP and creatine phosphate concentrations. Some of the sensitized animals died within an observation period of 24 hours following the isoproterenol injection. Their hearts exhibited infarct-like, confluent necrotic areas.

The intracellular sites where the splitting of ATP is activated by excess Ca are probably situated in different structures. Evidence exists that, in addition to the myofibrils and the sarcoplasmic reticulum, the mitochondria also participate in the high-energy phosphate breakdown. It is a well known fact that isolated mitochondria from heart muscle[47] as well as from liver, kidney or suprarenal cortex*) can rapidly concentrate Ca by means of an ATP-driven active transport system while the rate of oxygen uptake rises. But with increasing binding of Ca the mitochondria are badly damaged both morphologically and in relation to their biochemical function since they swell and deteriorate in their respiratory control and phosphorylating capacity. In this way intracellular excess Ca can also inhibit ATP synthesis in addition to enhancing ATP consumption. The fatal Ca-induced loss of high-energy phosphates leading to cardiac necrotization is probably due to a combination of these two effects. Therefore it is not surprising that similar changes to those produced in isolated

---

*Concerning the Ca effects on liver mitochondria, see Rossi and Lehninger,[48] Carafoli and Rossi,[5] Azzi and Azzone,[2] and Cohn et al.[7] Similar results with Ca were obtained on kidney mitochondria by Cohn et al.[6] and on mitochondria from suprarenal cortex by Whysner et al.[56]

mitochondria, suspended in a medium with excess Ca, were found in mitochondria from isoproterenol-treated rat hearts. Here, too, the mitochondria were considerably swollen, and respiratory control was impaired.[53]

All these observations justify the conclusion that the crucial point in the catecholamine-induced destruction of heart muscle is an abundant Ca influx, a state of excitation-contraction 'over-coupling' in which the myocardial fibres are killed if they cannot get rid of the Ca overload. In other words, the excessive intracellular Ca uptake must be considered to be the determinant factor in the etiology of catecholamine-induced myocardial fibre necroses rather than a concomitant or subsequent phenomenon.

References

1. Antoni, H., Engstfeld, G. and Fleckenstein, A. (1960). Inotrope Effekte von ATP und Adrenalin am hypodynamen Froschmyokard nach elektro-mechanischer Entkoppelung durch Ca^{++}-Entzug. Pflüg. Arch. ges. Physiol., **272**, 91.

2. Azzi, A. and Azzone, G. F. (1966). Swelling and shrinkage phenomena in liver mitochondria: III. Irreversible swelling induced by inorganic phosphate and Ca^{2+}. Biochim. biophys. acta, **113**, 438.

3. Bajusz, E. (1963). 'Conditioning Factors for Cardiac Necroses'. Karger, Basel and New York.

4. Byon, Y. K. and Fleckenstein, A. (1969). Parallelism between isometric tension and oxygen consumption of isolated papillary muscles under the influence of Ca ions, adrenaline, isoproterenol and organic Ca antagonists (Iproveratril, D600, Prenylamine). Pflüg. Arch. ges. Physiol., **312**, R8.

5. Carafoli, E. and Rossi, C. S. (1967). Ca^{++}-dependent movements of H^+ and K^+ across the rat liver mitochondrial membrane. Europ. J. Biochem., **2**, 224.

6. Cohn, D. V., Bawdon, R. and Eller, G. (1967). The effect of parathyroid hormone in vivo on the accumulation of calcium and phosphate by kidney and on kidney mitochondrial function. J. biol. Chem., **242**, 1253.

7. Cohn, D. V., Bawdon, R., Newman, R. R. and Hamilton, J. W. (1968). Effect of calcium chelation on the ion content of liver mitochondria in carbon tetrachloride-poisoned rats. J. biol. Chem., **243**, 1089.

8. Ebashi, S. and Lipmann, F. (1962). Adenosine triphosphate-linked concentration of calcium ions in a particulate fraction of rabbit muscle. J. Cell biol., **14**, 389.

9   Fanburg, B., Finkel, R.M. and Martonosi, A. (1964). The role of calcium in the mechanism of relaxation of cardiac muscle. J.biol.Chem., **239**, 2298.

10 Fleckenstein, A. (1963). Metabolic aspects of the excitation-contraction coupling. In 'Symposium on the Cellular Function of Membrane Transport', 16th Annual Meeting of the Society of General Physiologists, Woods Hole, Mass., September 1963. Hoffman, J.F. (Ed.). Prentice-Hall, Englewood Cliffs, New Jersey.

11 Fleckenstein, A. (1964). Die Bedeutung der energiereichen Phosphate für Kontraktilität und Tonus des Myokards. Verh. dtsch.Ges. inn.Med., **70**, 81.

12 Fleckenstein, A. (1968a). Experimentelle Pathologie der akuten und chronischen Herzinsuffizienz. Ferh.dtsch.Ges. KreislForsch., **34**, 15.

13 Fleckenstein, A. (1968b). Myokardstoffwechsel und Nekrose. In 'VI Symposium der Deutsch. Ges. für Fortschritte auf dem Gebiet der Inneren Medizin über "Herzinfarkt und Schock"', Freiburg, November 1968. Heilmeyer, L. and Holtmeier, H.-J. (Eds.), pp. 94-109. Georg Thieme Verlag, Stuttgart.

14 Fleckenstein, A. (in press). Pathophysiologische, Kausalfaktoren bei Myokard-Nekrose und Infarkt: 14. Kardio-angiologische Diskussion der Österreichischen Kardiologischen Gesellschaft, Wien, November 1969.

15 Fleckenstein, A., Döring, H.J. and Kammermeier, H. (1967). Experimental heart failure due to inhibition of utilisation of high-energy phosphates. In 'International Symposium on the Coronary Circulation and Energetics of the Myocardium', Milan, 1966, pp. 220-236. Karger, Basel and New York.

16 Fleckenstein, A., Döring, H.J. and Kammermeier, H. (1968). Einfluss von Beta-Receptorenblockern und Verwandten Substanzen auf Erregung, Kontraktion und Energiestoffwechsel der Myokardfaser. Klin.Wschr., **46**, 343.

17 Fleckenstein, A., Döring, H.J. and Leder, O. (1969). The significance of high-energy phosphate exhaustion in the etiology of isoproterenol-induced cardiac necroses and its prevention by iproveratril, compound D600 or prenylamine. In 'Symposium International on Drugs and Metabolism of Myocardium and Striated Muscle'. Lamarche, M. and Royer, R. (Eds.), Nancy.

18 Fleckenstein, A., Kammermeier, H., Döring, H.J. and Freund, H.J. (1967). Zum Wirkungsmechanismus neuartiger Koronardilatatoren mit gleichzeitig Sauerstoffeinsparenden Myokard-Effekten, Prenylamin und Iproveratril. Z. KreislForsch., **56**, 716.

19 Fleckenstein, A., Tritthart, H., Fleckenstein, B., Herbst, A. and Grün, G. (1969). Eine neue Gruppe kompetitiver Ca^{++}-Antagonisten (Iproveratril, D600, Prenylamin) mit starken Hemmeffekten auf die elektromechanische Koppelung im Warmblüter-Myokard. Pflüg. Arch. ges. Physiol., **307**, 25.

20 Gersmeyer, G. and Holland, W.C. (1963). Influence of ouabain on contractile force, resting tension, Ca^{45} entry and tissue Ca content in rat atria. Circ. Res., **12**, 620.

21 Grossman, A. and Furchgott, R.F. (1965). The effects of various drugs on calcium exchange in the isolated guinea-pig left auricle. J. Pharmacol., **145**, 162.

22 Haas, H. and Busch, E. (1967). Vergleichende Untersuchungen der Wirkung von α-Isopropyl-α-((N-methyl-N-homoveratryl)-γ-aminopropyl)-3,4-dimethoxyphenylacetonitril, seiner Derivate sowie einiger anderer Coronardilatatoren und β-Receptor-affiner Substanzen. Arzneimittelforsch., **17**, 257.

23 Haas, H. and Härtfelder, G. (1962). α-Isopropyl-α-((N-methyl-N-homoveratryl)-γ-aminopropyl)-3,4-dimethoxyphenylacetonitril, eine Substanz mit coronargefässerweiternden Eigenschaften. Arzneimittelforsch., **12**, 549.

24 Hanforth, C.P. (1962). Isoproterenol-induced myocardial infarction in animals. Arch. Path., **73**, 161.

25 Hasselbach, W. and Makinose, M. (1961). Die Ca^{++}-Pumpe der Erschlaffungsgrana des Muskels und ihre Abhängigkeit von der ATP-Spaltung. Biochem. Z., **333**, 518.

26 Herrell, W.E. (1967). Beer and cobalt and cardiohepatic failure. Clin. Med., **74**, 15.

27 Holland, W.C. and Sekul, A. (1958). Effect of ouabain on Ca^{45} and Cl^{36} exchange in isolated rabbit atria. Amer. J. Physiol., **197**, 757.

28 Jaedicke, W., Janke, J. and Fleckenstein, A. (1970). Potentiation of isoproterenol-induced cardiac necrosis by augmentation of transmembrane Ca influx with the use of 9-α-fluorocortisol acetate — neutralization of this effect by K or Mg salts. Pflüg. Arch. ges. Physiol., **319**, R9.

29 Janke, J., Fleckenstein, A. and Jaedicke, W. (1970). Inhibition of the isoproterenol-induced radiocalcium uptake into the ventricular myocardium by Ca-antagonistic inhibitors of excitation-contraction coupling (Isoptin = verapamil, iproveratril or compound D600). Pflüg. Arch. ges. Physiol., **316**, R10.

30 Janke, J., Jaedicke, W. and Fleckenstein, A. (1970). Prevention of isoproterenol-induced cardiac necrosis by reduction of transmembrane Ca influx with the use of K and Mg salts or of Ca-antagonistic inhibitors of excitation-contraction coupling. Pflüg. Arch. ges. Physiol., **319**, R8.

31 Kammermeier, H. (1964). Verhalten von Adenin-Nucleotiden und Kreatinphosphat im Herzmuskel bei funktioneller Erholung nach länger dauernder Asphyxie. Verh. dtsch. Ges. KreislForsch., **30**, 206.

32 Kammermeier, H. and Döring, H.J. (1961). Eine neue Methode zur fortlaufenden, direktschreibenden Registreirung des Mechanogramms sowie der Dilatation am freigelegten Herzen im Tierexperiment. Wegmessung mit tastlosen induktiven Aufnehmern. Pflüg. Arch. ges. Physiol., **273**, 311.

33 Katz., A.M. (1970). Contractile proteins of the heart. Physiol. Rev., **50**, 63.

34   Kaufmann, R. and Fleckenstein, A. (1965). Ca^{++}-competitive elektro-mechanische Entkoppelung durch Ni^{++}- und Co^{++}-Ionen am Warmblutermyokard. Pflüg. Arch. ges. Physiol., **282**, 290.

35   Klaus, W. and Lee, K S. (1969). Influence of cardiac glycosides on calcium binding in muscle subcellular components. J. Pharmacol., **166**, 68.

36   Lee, K.S., Hong, Sa.A. and Kang, D.H. (1970). Effect of cardiac glycosides on interaction of Ca with mitochondria. J. Pharmacol., **172**, 180.

37   Lindner, E. (1960). Phenyl-propyl-diphenyl-propyl-amin, eine neue Substanz mit coronargefässerweiternder Wirkung. Arzneimittelforsch., **10**, 569.

38   Lindner, E. (1961). Wirkung von N-(3-Phenyl-propyl-(2))-1,1-diphenyl-propyl-(3)-amin Glutonat auf den Herzmuskelstoffwechsel. Verh. dtsch. Ges. KreislForsch., **27**, 256.

39   Loewi, O. (1917). Über den Zusammenhang zwischen Digitalis- und Calciumwirkung. Naunyn-Schmiedebergs Arch. exp. Path. Pharmakol., **82**, 131.

40   Lüllmann, H. and Holland, W.C. (1962). Influence of ouabain on an exchangeable calcium fraction, contractile force, and resting tension of guinea-pig atria. J. Pharmacol., **137**, 186.

41   Raab, W. (1963). Neurogenic multifocal destruction of myocardial tissue. Rev. canad. Biol., **22**, 217.

42   Reuter, H. (1965). Über die Wirkung von Adrenalin auf den cellulären Ca-Umsatz des Meerschweinchenvorhofs. Naunyn-Schmiedebergs Arch. exp. Path. Pharmakol., **251**, 401.

43   Rona, G., Chappel, C.I., Balazs, T. and Gaudry, R. (1959) An infarct-like myocardial lesion and other toxic manifestations produced by isoproterenol in the rat. A.M.A. Arch. Path., **67**, 443.

44 Rona, G., Chappel, C.I. and Kahn, D.S. (1963). The significance of factors modifying the development of isoproterenol-induced myocardial necrosis. Amer. Heart J., **66**, 389.

45 Rona, G., Kahn, D.S. and Chappel, C.I. (1963). Studies on infarct-like myocardial necrosis produced by isoproterenol: A review. Rev. canad. Biol., **22**, 241.

46 Rosenblum, I., Wohl, A. and Stein, A. (1965). Studies in cardiac necrosis. III. Metabolic effects of sympathomimetic amines producing cardiac lesions. Toxicol. appl. Pharmacol., **7**, 344.

47 Rosenmann, E., Gazenfield, E., Laufer, A. and Davies, A.M. (1964). Isoproterenol-induced myocardial lesions in the immunized and nonimmunized rat. Path. microbiol. (Basel), **27**, 303.

48 Rossi, C.S. and Lehninger, A.L. (1964). Stoichiometry of respiratory stimulation, accumulation of Ca^{++} and phosphate and oxidative phosphorylation in rat liver mitochondria. J. biol. Chem., **239**, 3971.

49 Schildberg, F.W. and Fleckenstein, A. (1965). Die Bedeutung der extracellulären Calciumkonzentration für die Spaltung von energiereichem Phosphat in ruhendem und tätigem Myokardgewebe. Pflüg. Arch. ges. Physiol., **283**, 137.

50 Sekul, A. and Holland, W.C. (1960). Effects of ouabain on Ca^{45} entry in quiescent and electrically driven rabbit atria. Amer. J. Physiol., **199**, 457.

51 Selye, H. (1960). 'Elektrolyte, Stress und Herznekrose'. Benno Schwabe, Basel.

52 Slater, E.C. and Cleland, K.W. (1953). The effect of calcium on the respiratory and phosphorylative activities of heart-muscle sarcosomes. Biochem. J., **55**, 566.

53 Stanton, H.C. and Schwartz, A. (1967). Effects of a hydrazine monoamine oxidase inhibitor (phenelzine) on isoproterenol-induced myocardiopathies in the rat. J. Pharmacol., **157**, 649.

54 Sullivan, J.F., Egan, J.D., George, R.P. and McDermott, P.M. (1966). Cardiohepatic failure in beer drinkers. Proc. cent. Soc. clin. Res., **39**, 138.

55 Thomas, L.J., Jolley, W.B. and Grechman, R. (1958). Effect of potassium lack and ouabain on calcium^{45} uptake in frog's heart. Fed. Proc., **17**, 162.
(See Thomas, L.J. (1960). Ouabain contracture of frog heart: Ca^{45} movements and effect of EDTA. Amer. J. Physiol., **199**, 146.)

56 Whysner, J.A., Paule, W.J., Nelson, D.H. and Harding, B.W. (1966). The mechanism of calcium effects on steroid biosynthesis by adrenal mitochondria. Clin. Res., **14**, 180.

AUTHOR INDEX

Allen, J.C., 18(5), **19**, 87(2, 22), **90**, **91**, 110(1), **115**
Antoni, H., 47(1), **56**, 156(1), **182**
Aronson, C.E., 98(43), **119**
Azzi, A., 106(71, 79), **121**, **122**, 180(2), **182**
Azzone, G.F., 106(71, 80), 109(72), **121**, **122**, 180(2), **182**

Bachmann, E., 108(5, 6), **115**
Bailey, K., 10(1), **19**
Bajusz, E., 89(19), **91**, 173(3), **182**
Baker, H., 4(39), 5(39), **22**
Balazs, T., 157(43), **186**
Banga, I., 4(2), 6(2), **19**
Bárány, M., 4(3), **19**, 130(1), **134**
Baum, H., 106(37), **118**
Bawdon, R., 180(6, 7), **182**
Beeler, G.W., Jr., 35(2, 3), 46(2, 3), 47(3), **56**
Behnke, O., 33(81), 44(81), **63**
Bendall, J.R., 8(4), **19**, 69(1), **90**
Bennett, H.S., 31(4), **56**
Benson, E.S., 31(56), 43(56, 91), **61**, **64**
Bertaud, W.S., 31(73), **62**
Besch, H.R., Jr., 18(5), **19**, 87(2), **90**, 110(1, 2), **115**
Bianchi, C.P., 3(6), **19**, **56**
Bielawski, J., 109(3), **115**
Blaustein, M.P., 47(6), **56**
Blinks, J.R., 40(33), **59**
Blum, J.J., 10(41), **22**
Botts, J., 10(41), **22**
Bozler, E., 8(7), **19**
Brady, A.J., 28(38), 39(38), 45(38), **59**, 67(3), **90**
Breeman, C. van, 52(92), **64**

Bresnick, E., 68(4), 72(4), **90**
Bretschneider, H.J., 102(44, 63), 103(4), **115**, **119**, **121**
Brierley, G.P., 108(5, 6, 7), **115**
Briggs, F.N., **17**(8, 17, 34), **19**, **20**, **22**, 25(19), 50(34), 52(20), **57**, **59**, 112(42), **119**
Brunton, K., 100(8), **115**
Busch, E., 143(22), **184**
Byon, Y.K., 149(4), 154(4), 155(4), **182**

Caldwell, P.C., 25(72), **62**
Caplan, A., 108(9), **115**
Carafoli, E., 15(48), **23**, 97(54, 62), 98(62), 102(22), 105(14), 106(12, 54), 108(9, 10, 11, 16, 53), 109(13, 15, 22, 54), **115**, **116**, **117**, **120**, 180(5), **182**
Carlson, F.D., 24(7), **56**
Carmeliet, E., 54(8), **56**
Carson, V., 52(54, 55), **60**
Carsten, M.E., 15(9), **19**
Chance, B., 97(18), 106(17, 59), 108(59), 109(58, 66), **116**, **120**, **121**
Chapell, J.B., 108(20), 109(19, 20), **116**
Chappel, C.I., 157(43), 173(44), **186**, **187**
Chipperfield, D., 52(54, 55), **60**
Choi, S.J., 17(37), **22**, 45(40), **59**
Christianson, R.O., 109(21), **117**
Cleland, K.W., **187**
Cohn, D.V., 180(6, 7), **182**
Conover, T.E., 4(3), **19**
Constantin, L.L., 33(9), **56**
Coraboeuf, E., 35(10), **57**
Cranefield, P.F., 35(26), **58**
Crofts, A.R., 109(19), **116**

Crow, C., 89(19), **91**

Daile, P., 52(55), **60**
Davies, A.M., 161(47), 180(47), **187**
Davies, R.E., 10(10), **19**, 24(11), **57**
DeLuca, H.F., **121, 122**
Dhalla, N.S., 17(43), **22**, 102(60), **120**
Ditmer, D.S., 25(12), **57**
Döring, H.J., 136(15, 16, 18), 141(18), 149(15, 16, 32), 151(15, 16, 18), 153(15), 156(15), 157(17), 158(17), 161(17), 167(17), **183, 184, 185**
Drahota, Z., 102(22, 24), 106(23), 109(22), **117**
Dransfeld, H., 110(25, 26, 27), 111(25), **117**

Eadie, G.S., 99(28), 100(28), **117**
Ebashi, F., 11(11, 13), **20**, 101(30), **117**
Ebashi, S., 8(33), 9(14), 10(12), 11(11, 12, 13), **20, 21**, 25(13), **57**, 69(6, 7), 70(7), 75(6, 12), 76(12, 21), 85(5), **90, 91**, 95(29, 31, 45, 50), 101(30), **117, 118, 119**, 138(8), **182**
Edman, K.A., 132(2), **134**
Egan, J.D., 141(54), **188**
Eller, G., 180(6), **182**
Endo, M., 25(13), **57**, 69(6), 75(6), **90**
Engelhardt, A., 4(15), **20**
Engstfeld, G., 156(1), **182**
Entman, M.L., 52(14), 54(15), **57**, 112(32), **118**
Epstein, S.E., 52(14), 54(15), **57**, 112(32), **118**

Ernster, L., 106(23, 33), **117, 118**

Fahrenbach, W.H., 33(16), 45(16), 52(16), **57**
Fanburg, B., 95(34), **118**, 138(9), **183**
Fang, M., **121**
Farah, A., 40(80), 48(80), **63**
Fawcett, D.W., 31(17), 33(17), **57**
Fehmers, M.C.O., 98(35), **118**
Feretos, R., 45(44), **60**
Finkel, R.M., 95(34), **118**, 138(9), **183**
Fleckenstein, A., 15(16), **20**, 136(10, 15, 16, 18, 49), 141(18, 34), 143(11, 12, 19), 149(4, 11, 15, 16), 150(11), 151(11, 15, 16, 18), 153(15), 154(4), 155(4), 156(1, 15), 157(13, 17), 158(17), 160(13), 161(13, 17), 165(13), 166(14, 28, 29, 30), 167(17), **183, 184, 185, 186, 187**
Fleckenstein, B., 143(19), **184**
Forssmann, W.G., 31(18), 33(18), **57**
Frank, G.B., 66(8), **90**
Franzen, J., 4(42), **22**
Franzini-Armstrong, C., 33(9), **56**
Freund, H.J., 136(18), 141(18), 151(18), **184**
Fuchs, F., 25(19), **57**
Furchgott, R.F., 3(20), **20**, 37(22), 48(23), 52(22), **58**, 156(21), **184**

Gaetjens, E., 4(3), **19**
Gamble, R.L., 102(22), 109(13, 22), **116, 117**
Gaudry, R., 157(43), **186**

AUTHOR INDEX

Gazenfield, E., 161(47), 180(47), 187
Gear, A.R.L., 109(36), **118**
George, R.P., 141(54), **188**
Gergely, J., 128(3), **134**
Gersmeyer, G., 156(20), **184**
Gertz, E.W., 17(8, 17, 34), 18(18), **19, 20, 22**, 50(34), 52(20), **57, 59**
Girardier, L., 31(18), 33(18), **57**
Glick, G., 18(5), **19**, 87(2), **90**, 110(1), **115**
Glynn, I., 18(19), **20**
Goffart, M., 4(3), **19**
Govier, W.C., 52(21), **58**
Greaser, M.L., 128(3), **134**
Grebe, D., 102(63), **121**
Grebe, R.M., 25(12), **57**
Grechman, R., 156(55), **188**
Greeff, K., 110(26, 27), **117**
Green, D.E., 106(37), 108(5, 6, 7), **115, 118**
Greenawalt, J.W., 109(86), **123**
Greville, G.D., 108(20), 109(20), **116**
Grey, T.C., 8(49), 11(50), **23**
Grossman, A., 3(20), **20**, 37(22), 48(23), 52(22), **58**, 156(21), **184**
Grün, G., 143(19), **184**

Haas, H., 143(22, 23), **184**
Hamer, J., 112(42, 82, 84), **119, 122, 123**
Hamilton, J.W., 180(7), **182**
Hanforth, C.P., 157(24), 177(24), **184**
Hansen, J., 6(28), **21**
Harding, B.W., 180(56), **188**

Harigaya, S., 17(21), **20**, 76(9), 79(9), 87(9, 22), 89(19), **90, 91**, 97(38), 101(38), 105(38), **118**
Harris, E.J., 40(62), **61**
Härtfelder, G., 143(23), **184**
Hartshorne, D.J., 12(22, 23, 24), **21**, 25(24), **58**, 128(4), **134**
Hasselbach, W., 9(25), **21**, 33(25), **58**, 73(10), 74(10), **90**, 95(39, 61), **118, 120**, 138(25), **185**
Haugaard, E.S., 97(40), 98(41), 106(40), **118**
Haugaard, N.N., 97(40), 98(41, 43), 106(40), **118, 119**
Hecht, H.A., 85(14), **91**
Heilbrun, L.V., 3(26), **21**
Heppner, R.L., 46(101), 47(101), 48(101), **65**
Herbst, A., 143(19), **184**
Herrell, W.E., 141(26), **185**
Herz, R·, 15(55), **23**, 24(95), 25(95), 39(94), **64**, 72(25, 26), **92**, 95(88, 90), 97(89), **123**
Hess, D., 110(26), **117**
Hess, M.L., 17(8, 17, 34), **19, 20, 22**, 50(34), 52(20), **57, 59**, 98, 112(42, 43, 82), **119, 122**
Hill, A.V., 129(5), **134**
Hill, T.L., 10(41), **22**
Hodgkin, A.L., 47(6), **56**
Hoffman, B.F., 35(26), **58**
Holland, W.C., 40(82), 52(21, 42, 82), **58, 59, 63**, 156(20, 27, 40, 50), 173(40), **184, 185, 186, 187**
Hong, Sa.A., 156(36), **186**
Honig, C.R., 69(11), **91**
Horn, R.S., 97(40), 98(41, 43), 106(40), **118, 119**
Howell, J.N., 33(68), **62**

Hübner, G., 102(44, 63), **119, 121**
Huxley, A. F., 6(27), **21**, 24(27), 44(27, 29), **58**, 132(6), **134**
Huxley, H. E., 6(28), 7(29), 12(29), **21**, 24(28), **58**

Inesi, G., 75(12), 76(12), **91**, 95(45, 65), **119, 121**

Jacob, R., 47(1), **56**
Jaedicke, W., 166(28, 29, 30), **185**
Janke, J., 166(28, 29, 30), **185**
Jenden, D. J., 33(68), **62**
Jolley, W. B., 156(55), **188**

Kahn, D. S., 173(44), **187**
Kammermeier, H., 136(15, 16, 18), 141(18), 149(15, 16, 32), 151(15, 16, 18), 153(15), 156(15), 166(31), **183, 184, 185**
Kang, D. H., 156(36), **186**
Kaninga, Z., 106(85), **123**
Karnovsky, M. J., 28(78), **63**
Kasuya, Y., 45(40), **59**
Katz, A. M., 15(30), **21**, 24(30), 39(31), 45(31), **58**, 69(13), 85(14), 87(13), **91**, 95(46), 97(46), **119**, 124(7), 127(7), 132(7), **134** 138(33), **185**
Kaufmann, R., 47(1), **56**, 141(34), **186**
Kavaler, F., 46(32), **58**
Kielley, W. W., 8(31), **21**
Klaus, W., 156(35), **186**
Koch-Weser, J., 40(33), **59**

Kodama, A., 10(12), 11(12, 13), **20**, 101(30), **117**
Koller, H., 43(97), **64**
Kostrzewa, R., 98(41), **118**
Kübler, W., 15(32), **21**, 102(47, 48, 49), 103(47), **119**
Kumagai, H., 8(33), **21**, 95(50), **119**

Ladinsky, H., 17(36), **22**, 45(40), **59**
Lain, R. F., 17(17, 34), **20, 22**, 50(34), 52(20), **57, 59**
Langer, G. A., 3(35), **22**, 24(37), 27(35), 28(38, 86), 31(37), 37(35), 39(35, 38), 40(36, 37, 39), 45(38), 47(35), 52(39), **59, 63**, 101(51), **119**
Laufer, A., 161(47), 180(47), **187**
Leder, O., 157(17), 158(17), 161(17), 167(17), **184**
Lee, C.-P., 106(33), **118**
Lee, K. S., 17(36, 37), **22**, 45(40), **59**, 75(15), **91**, 156(35, 36), **186**
Lee, N. H., 97(40), 98(41), 106(40), **118**
Lehninger, A. L., 97(54), 99(70), 102(22, 24), 105(14), 106(54, 70), 107(70), 108(16, 52, 53, 70, 73), 109(3, 13, 15, 22, 36, 54, 73, 74), **115, 116, 117, 118, 120, 121, 122**, 180(48), **187**
Levy, G. S., 52(14), 54(15), **57**, 112(32), **118**
Lindner, E., 143(37), **186**
Lipmann, F., 9(14), **20**, 69(7), 70(7), **90**, 95(31), **118**, 138(8), **182**
Ljubimova, J., 4(15), **20**
Locke, F. S., 2(38), **22**, 25(41), **59**
Lodinsky, H., 17(36), **22**

AUTHOR INDEX

Loewi, O., 156(39), **186**
Lowey, S., 4(39), 5(39), **22**
Loyter, A., 109(21), **117**
Lüllmann, H., 52(42), **59,** 156 (40), 173(40), **186**
Luttgau, H.C., 43(43), **59,** 66 (16, 17), **91**

Makinose, M., 9(25), **21,** 73(10), 74(10), **90,** 95(39, 61), **118, 120,** 138(25), **185**
Marsh, B.B., 7(40), **22,** 67(18), **91**
Martonosi, A., 45(44), **60,** 95 (34), **118,** 138(9), **183**
Mascher, D., 35(45), **60**
McCollum, W.B., 89(19), **91**
McDermott, P.M., 141(54), **188**
McInnes, I., 52(55), **60**
McIntosh, D.A.D., 45(85), **63,** 112(78), **122**
McNaughton, C., 52(92), **64**
McNutt, N.S., 31(17), 33(17), **57**
Mela, L., 105(57), 106(55, 56, 57, 59), 108(57, 59), 109(58), **120**
Merrillees, N.C.R., 43(53), **60**
Meyerhof, O., 8(31), **21**
Mines, G.R., 25(46), **60**
Mommaerts, W.F.H.M., 69 (23), **91**
Morad, M., 46(47), **60**
Morales, M.F., 10(41), **22**
Mueller, H., 4(42), 12(22, 23), **21, 22,** 25(24), **58,** 128(4), **134**
Muir, J.R., 17(43, 44), **22,** 102 (60), **120**
Muller, P., 44(48), **60**

Murer, E., 108(6, 7), **115**

Nagai, T., 95(61), **120**
Nayler, W.G., 3(45), **23,** 27(49, 50, 51), 37(51), 40(51), 43(53), 52(52, 54, 55), **60**
Nelson, D.A., 31(56), 43(56), **61**
Nelson, D.H., 180(56), **188**
Newman, R.R., 180(7), **182**
Niedergerke, R., 3(46), 6(27), **21, 23,** 24(60), 27(59), 35(63), 37(61), 40(57, 59, 61, 62), 41(59), 43(43), **59, 61,** 66(17), 67(20), **91**
Nierop, C. van, 69(11), **91**
Nilsson, E., 132(2), **134**

Oertelis, S.J., 31(89), 44(89), **64**
Ogata, E., 108(67), 109(66), **121**
Ohnishi, T., 76(21), **91**
Olson, R.E., 4(42), 15(47), 17(43, 44), **22, 23,** 102(60), **120**
Orkand, R.F., 35(63), 40(64), **61**
Orteza, J.M., 17(43), **22,** 102(60), **120**

Page, E., 31(65), 44(65), **61**
Palmer, R.F., 45(66), **61**
Park, J.K., 105(64), **121**
Patriarca, P., 15(48), **23,** 97(62), 98(62), **120**
Paule, W.J., 180(56), **188**
Paulussen, F., 102(44, 63), **119, 121**
Peachey, L.D., 33(67), **61**
Pease, D.C., 33(68), **62**
Peper, K., 35(45), **60**
Perry, S.V., 8(49), 11(50), **23**
Podolsky, R.J., 25(69), 33(9), **56, 62,** 132(9), **134**
Pohl, W.G., 95(65), **121**

Pool, P.E., 24(70), **62**
Porter, K.R., 31(4, 71), **56, 62**
Portzehl, H., 25(72), **62**
Posey, V.A., 45(66), **61**
Pressman, B.C., 105(64), **121**
Pretorius, P.J., 95(65), **121**

Raab, W., 161(41), **186**
Racker, E., 109(21), **117**
Rasmussen, H., 108(67), 109 (66), **121, 122**
Rayns, D.G., 31(73), 33(90), **62, 64**
Reiss, I., 15(55), **23**, 24(95), 25 (95), **64**, 72(25, 26), **92**, 95(88, 90), 97(89), **123**
Repke, D.I., 15(30), **21**, 39(31), 45(31), **58**, 95(46), 97(46), **119**
Reuter, H., 35(2, 3, 74, 75, 76), 46(2, 3), 47(3, 77), **56, 62**, 95 (69), **121**, 156(42), **186**
Revel, J.P., 28(78), **63**
Reynafarje, B., 99(70), 106(70), 107(70), 108(70), 109(36), **118, 121**
Rice, R.V., 4(42), **22**
Ringer, S., 2(51), **23**, 25(79), 40 (79), **63**
Rona, G., 157(43), 173(44), **186, 187**
Rosenblum, I., 161(46), **187**
Rosenheim, O., 2(38), **22**, 25(41), **59**
Rosenmann, E., 161(47), 180 (47), **187**
Rosin, H., 40(80), 48(80), **63**
Rossi, C.S., 97(54), 102(22), 105(14), 106(54, 71), 108(73), 109(13, 15, 22, 36, 54, 72, 73, 74), **116, 117, 118, 120, 121, 122**, 180(5, 48), **182, 187**

Rostgaard, J., 33(81), 44(81), **63**
Ruegg, J.C., 25(72), **62**

Sabatini-Smith, S., 40(82), 52(82), **63**
Sallis, J.D., **121, 122**
Saltzgaber, J., 109(21), **117**
Sanadi, D.R., 106(76), **122**
Sandow, A., 24(84), 27(83, 84), **63**
Saris, N.E., 109(77), **122**
Scales, B., 45(85), **63**, 112(78), **122**
Scarpa, A., 106(79, 80), **122**
Scatchard, G., 98(81), 99(81), 106 (81), 107(81), **122**
Schildberg, F.W., 136(49), **187**
Schliselfeld, L.H., 4(3), **19**
Scholz, H., 35(76), **62**, 95(69), **121**
Schorn, A., 110(26, 27), **117**
Schwartz, A., 17(21), 18(5), **19, 20**, 68(4), 72(4), 76(9), 79(9), 87(2, 9, 22), 89(19), **90, 91**, 97(38), 101 (38), 105(38), 110(1, 2), **115, 118**, 157(53), 181(53), **187**
Schwartz, W.B., 15(47), **23**
Sekul, A., 156(27, 50), **185, 187**
Selye, H., 173(51), **187**
Serena, S.D., 28(86), 40(39), 52 (39), **59, 63**
Shanes, A.M., 3(6, 57), **19, 23**, 27 (100), 37(100), 38(100), **65**
Shelburne, J.C., 28(86), **63**
Shinebourne, E.A., 15(32), **21**, 52 (87), 54(87), **63**, 112(42, 82, 83, 84, 91), **122, 123**
Sietz, H., 47(77), **62**
Simpson, F.O., 31(73, 88, 89), 33 (88, 90), 44(89), **62, 63, 64**
Slater, E.C., 106(85), **123, 187**
Slayter, H.S., 4(39), 5(39), **22**
Smithen, C.S., 95(65), **121**

Sonnenblick, E.H., 18(18), **20**, 24(70), **62**, 132(8), **134**
Spieckermann, P.G., 102(44), **119**
Staley, N.A., 43(91), **64**
Stam, A.C., 18(18), **20**
Stanton, H.C., 157(53), 181(53), **187**
Steensland, H., 109(21), **117**
Stein, A., 161(46), **187**
Stone, J., 52(54), **60**
Stuckey, J.H., 17(36), **22**
Sullivan, J.F., 141(54), **188**
Szent-Gyorgi, A., 4(2), 6(2), **19**

Takeda, F., 8(33), **21**, 95(50), **119**
Taylor, R.E., 44(29), **58**
Teichholz, L.E., 132(9), **134**
Theiner, M., 12(23), **21**, 128(4), **134**
Thomas, L.J., 156(55), **188**
Ting, B.T., 110(27), **117**
Trautwein, W., 46(47), **60**
Tritthart, H., 143(19), **184**

Uchida, K., 69(23), **91**

Vasington, F.D., 109(86), **123**

Vereecke, J., 54(8), **56**

Watanabe, S., 8(52), **23**, 75(12), 76(12), **91**, 95(45), **119**
Weber, A., 9(53), 11(54), 15(55), 17(44), **22**, **23**, 24(93, 95), 25(95), 39(94), **64**, 69(24), 71(24), 72(25, 26), 75(24), **92**, 95(88, 90), 97(89), 100(87), **123**
Weber, H.H., 4(56), **23**
Weeds, A.G., 4(39), 5(39), **22**
Weiland, S., 108(16), **116**
Weyne, J., 67(27), **92**
White, R., 52(87), 54(87), **63**, 112(82, 83, 84, 91), **122**, **123**
Whysner, J.A., 180(56), **188**
Wiedmann, S., 46(96, 101), 47(101), 48(101), **64**, **65**
Wiercinski, F.J., 3(26), **21**
Wilbrandt, W. von, 43(97), **64**
Winegrad, S., 3(57), **23**, 27(100), 37(100), 38(100), 40(98), **64**, **65**
Winicur, S., 11(54), **23**
Wohl, A., 161(46), **187**
Wojtczak, L., 106(85), **123**
Wood, E.H., 46(101), 47(101), 48(101), **65**

Young, R., **121**

SUBJECT INDEX

Actin, 4, 24
  polymerized, 6
  interaction with myosin, 85, 129
Action potential
  calcium exchange, associated with, 35-39
Actomyosin,
  activation by calcium, 125
  formation in muscle, 7
  reconstituted, 24
  saturation of, 39
  syneresis of, 84
  'synthetic', 11
Anoxia, 15, 17, 105, 161
Antagonistic drugs for calcium, types and effects, 141-181
Antifibrillatory drugs as calcium antagonists, 141
ATP,
  interchange with ADP, 73
  loss of, 166
  presence in myofibrils, 69
  splitting of, 73, 75, 180
ATP-ase activity, 4, 8, 11, 39, 71, 73, 125
  with myosin, 130
  maximal, requirement for, 138

Beating heart, 2-3
'Binding', 71
Blocking agents and drugs,
  effect on adrenaline, 54
  with antagonistic side effects, 141
Bodwitch staircase, 3

Cardiac failure, 2, 14-18
Contractile mechanism,
  excitation of, 14

Contractile proteins, 4-7, 125
  identification of, 2
Contractile system,
  activation of, 67
Contraction in heart muscle,
  activation of, 40-45
  membrane depolarization and, 46-54
Contraction-relaxation cycle, 8
  role of mitochondria, 98, 101, 105

Digitalis, 17
  effects of glycosides of, 156
  mechanism of action, 18
  in cardiac relaxing system, 87
  inotropic action of, 110

EDTA, inhibition by, 8, 11
Excitation-contraction coupling,
  alteration of action of, 18, 132
  substances for inhibition of, 141, 145-151
  theories of, 2-3, 10-15

F-actin, 6-7

G-actin, 6

Hyperlipidaemia, 161
Hypoxaemia, cardiac, 157
Hypoxia, 161
  accompanying ischaemia, 52

Inhibitors of calcium action, 135-150
Ischaemia, 52-161
  endocardial, 157

Lanthanide titration, technique, 108
Local anaesthetics,
 use as calcium antagonists, 141, 147
Longitudinal reticulum, 45

Membrane depolarization,
 effect on activation of contraction, 46-54
Meromyosin,
 heavy, 4
 light, 4
Michaelis-Menten equation, 100
Millipore filtration as assay method, 76
Mitochondria, 33, 93-114
 calcium accumulation by, 98, 105
 role in phosphate breakdown, 180
Myocardial cell,
 calcium activity in, 93-95
Myofibrils, 17
 diffusion into, 14
Myoplasm, 41-44
Myosin, 4, 24

Necrosis, cardiac, 161, 166
 disseminated, 169
 fibre, 173, 181

Phosphate consumption, high energy, 149, 157, 166
Phosphate deficiency, high energy, 157
Pinocytosis, 43
Promoters of calcium action, 151-156

Radiocalcium, uptake and accumulation, 173, 177
Radioisotope studies, 27
Relaxation, 7-9
 investigation of, 2
Relaxing factors, 7, 9, 69
 isolation of, 67
Relaxing system,
 binding constant, 80
 digitalis and, 87
 in failing heart, 87
 release phenomena and, 84
Release phenomena for calcium, 84

Sarcolemma, 28-30
 storage sites below, 44
Sarcomer, 6, 44
Sarcoplasm,
 removal of calcium from, 8
Sarcoplasmic reticulum, 31-33, 45
 associated cisternae, 31-33
 calcium uptake by, 66-90, 95, 112
 role in phosphate breakdown, 180
Spectrophotometry,
 dual beam method with murexide, 76
 stopped-flow methods, 76
'Staircase effect', 50
Superprecipitation, see Syneresis
Syneresis, of actomyosin, 85

Tracer experiments, 41
Transverse tubular system, 31
Tropomyosin, 10, 11
 complex with troponin, 128
 preparation of, 12

Troponin,
    affinity for, 80
    complex with tropomyosin, 128
    composition of, 12
    interaction with calcium, 125-133
    isolation of, 11
T system, 31

T tubules, diffusion through lumen, 44, 45
Trypsin, digestion of, 4

'Uptake', 71

Z band, 31
Z line, structure of, 7
Z tubules, 33

#216602

INT. STUDY GROUP FOR RE-
SEARCH...CALCIUM & THE
HEART   116620
WG202/1597C/70